Subhadra Menon has been a health and science writer for nearly two decades. As a print journalist, Menon was with the *India Today* magazine for five years. Before that she wrote for *Frontline*, *The New Scientist*, *Scientific American*, *Times of India*, *Economic Times* and *Indian Express*. She has also reported and written for BBC World and Reuters Health. She is the author of two books, *Buddhism* (*Classic India Series*) and *Trees of India*.

Menon holds a doctoral degree in reproductive ecology from the University of Delhi. She continues her work with the health sector in India. She is married and lives in Delhi with her husband and two children.

No Place to Go

Stories of Hope and Despair from India's
Ailing Health Sector

SUBHADRA   MENON

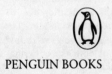

PENGUIN BOOKS

PENGUIN BOOKS

Published by the Penguin Group

Penguin Books India Pvt. Ltd, 11 Community Centre, Panchsheel Park, New Delhi 110 017, India

Penguin Group (USA) Inc., 375 Hudson Street, New York, NewYork 10014, USA

Penguin Group (Canada), 10 Alcorn Avenue, Toronto, Ontario, Canada M4V 3B2 (a division of Pearson Penguin Canada Inc.)

Penguin Books Ltd, 80 Strand, London WC2R 0RL, England

Penguin Ireland, 25 St Stephen's Green, Dublin 2, Ireland (a division of Penguin Books Ltd)

Penguin Group (Australia), 250 Camberwell Road, Camberwell, Victoria 3124, Australia (a division of Pearson Australia Group Pty Ltd)

Penguin Group (NZ), cnr Airborne and Rosedale Roads, Albany, Auckland 1310, New Zealand (a division of Pearson New Zealand Ltd)

Penguin Group (South Africa) (Pty) Ltd, 24 Sturdee Avenue, Rosebank, Johannesburg 2196, South Africa

Penguin Books Ltd, Registered Offices: 80 Strand, London WC2R 0RL, England

First published by Penguin Books India 2004

Copyright © Subhadra Menon 2004

Typeset in Sabon by Mantra Virtual Services, New Delhi
Printed at Sanat Printers, Kundli, Haryana

To Nayantara and Ashwat, for taking this in their stride

Contents

Acknowledgements

Some people say the germ of an idea is everything; the rest of the book follows automatically. It follows yes, but not without a lot of help, support, advice and cerebral inputs from so many people that one can lose count. This book is no different. When I first began to think about writing it, way back in 1999–2000, I approached it with very mixed feelings—anxiety, that the health sector was not delivering what it should to ordinary people, frustration, because there was so much infrastructure but it was not functional and was inaccessible to most people, and, most importantly, intense hope that if individuals and institutions got together to challenge the system and change it (and so many people were doing that already), there was no reason for it not to improve. Yet, all the resolve in the world would never have found tangible shape without the efforts of several people. I will try to acknowledge as many people as I can, but if I have forgotten to mention anyone, I request their pardon.

In the fifteen years that I have spent covering health as a print journalist in India, I have had the opportunity to work and write for some of the best magazines and newspapers of the country. I would like to thank Mr Aroon Purie, Editor-in-Chief, *India Today*, and Mr Raj Chengappa, Managing Editor, *India Today*, for giving me the opportunity to take some of India's burning health issues to the public and, in the process, learning intimately about the way the health sector functions, or malfunctions, in India. Mr K. Narayanan, former Deputy Editor, *Frontline*, was a major force in my early years as a journalist, allowing me the freedom to research and write about vital health issues that concern people across India.

Health journalism in India teaches you a lot of things—it becomes your magnifying glass to the way the health system functions in India, the problems and travails that people face while trying to access these services, the right and the wrong, the good and the bad. It brings you up close with people who are trying hard to make a difference either alone or through community-based experiments, small or big, and many of these efforts have meant the difference between life and death for several people. These years have taught me that the public health system also needs a revolution, much like the struggle to save the environment.

A lot of what is in this book has been vastly influenced by Professor V. Ramalingaswami, one of India's foremost medical professionals who made an enormous contribution to the public health sector, not just through his own work, but also by encouraging young people to understand the adversity in the field without losing sight of its strengths. I am also indebted to many others I met over the years—Dr Iqbal Malik, who worked tirelessly to put in systems for hospital waste management; Mr J.V.R. Prasada Rao, Secretary, Health, Ministry of Health and Family Welfare, who always found time for me and whose optimism is infectious; Professor Debabar Banerjee, Emeritus Scientist at the Jawaharlal Nehru University in New Delhi, whose writings and thoughts were always important catalysts; and Dr Naresh Trehan, Executive Director of the Escorts Heart Centre and Research Institute in New Delhi, whose patience in explaining the most complex of health issues will never give away the fact that he is among the busiest cardiac surgeons in the country today. I have over the years also drawn inspiration from Mr Jitendra Tuli, Mr K.S. Ahluwalia, Mr Ravi Duggal, Ms Neelam Krishnamoorthy, Mr Shekhar Krishnamoorthy, and Mr O.P. Sharma. I am thankful to Dr M. Venugopal for his patience and advice and to Dr Harsh Rastogi for always being there.

There are others who gave their valuable time whenever I asked for it—Dr K. Srinath Reddy, Chairman of the Department of Cardiology at the All India Institute of Medical Sciences, New Delhi; Dr C.P. Thakur, former Union Minister for Health and Family Welfare; and Professor N.K. Ganguly, Director General of the Indian Council of Medical Research. Many others were equally helpful: Dr K.K. Aggarwal, Dr M.S. Valiathan, Dr J.N. Pande, Dr Pradeep Seth, Mr S.R. Mohanty, Professor Ranjit Roy Chowdhury, Dr Prathap Reddy, Mr Suresh Guptan, Ms Tanuja Joshi, Dr P.V. Unnikrishnan, and Ms Geetanjali Chopra.

I would like to thank Professor H.V. Mohan Ram, Dr K.R. Shivanna and Professor C.R. Babu, my guides and mentors at the University of Delhi, who taught me the power of academic rigour and systematic research.

For nurturing an idea and shaping it into a book, I want to thank my editors at Penguin—Kamini Mahadevan, V.K. Karthika and Sonali Mukhopadhyay. All of us have friends who support us with no questions asked, who urge us to dream big, and who defy definition in terms of what their actual contribution to such an effort would be. I would like to thank Shammy Baweja, who always has a pragmatic solution for the most gigantic of problems, Saguna Dewan, for always being there, Tanuja Chaturvedi who will never say die, and Amita Bharath, who has always shared joys and sorrows. Many thanks to Ma and Amma. Also, thanks to Rema Raja for her generosity.

This book would not have been possible without Pallava,

my best friend and husband of many years. The writing of a book is such a time-intensive process that the patience with which he, and my two children, Nayantara and Ashwat, have stood by me through the process, has been remarkable. I hope I can do the same for them someday.

Introduction

India is the chosen land for millions across the world who seek spiritual well-being and peace. People come here from distant and remote places to attain, in their own modest way, spiritual wellness. It is the land where the Buddha attained nirvana, where Mahatma Gandhi lived and advocated a simple, rigorous and healthy life. It is now also the land of countless health resorts and wellness centres that have found their niches on the world tourism map. Excited travellers from across the globe come in search of sages and spirits, in search of real health solutions. It is the latest and 'hottest' dimension that the tourism industry has discovered, fuelling lucrative businesses—big and small—that run from diverse destinations in the Himalayas, the Western Ghats or anywhere along India's long and beautiful coastline. Health and health care make good business sense in the India of the present and the unique selling proposition of these businesses is that they offer packages that promise to take a person towards total health, through a holistic programme, which includes all the goodness of traditional Indian systems, the most popular being ayurveda, and combines it with the latest global programmes for healthy living. Energize your body and mind, say these centres over and over again, and for those of the easy spirit (with enough money too), these resorts are a great idea for a 'healthy' holiday.

For millions of Indians though, life is lived out very far from these resorts, and the distance is not just geographical. For them, life is a challenge because they have taken for granted their burden of diseases and disability, and the total erosion of the quality of their lives, believing that good health care is all too much to expect from the government, from the private sector, or from life in general. For them, luxury is not a spa, but to be able to hold in their arms a newborn child with the special knowledge that the mother of the baby is still alive; it is to manage to reach medical attention to an old parent in time to avoid death from a minor heart attack; it is to be safe after blood transfusion following a bad accident; it is to be able to get their children vaccinated against common, infectious diseases.

Is this then an embittered look at the haves and the have-nots, and have we not heard this before? Of course everybody has, but there is no bitterness here, only a realistic analysis of the health-care situation in India—what is in the package deal, and is it enough for the Indian on the street? Can he or she afford what is on offer, are there any discount packages, off-season deals? The comparisons drawn here are not to say that there is no inequity, but to highlight the irony of modern Indian society where health packages are offered to the healthy, but the procurement of basic, life-saving drugs and vaccines for the needy is the biggest challenge for the majority of people. The comparisons are drawn only to underscore the fact that inequity can be tolerated in all walks of life except health, and that there has to be a joint, social responsibility across the country to ensure that the health needs of the entire nation are not just addressed but also resolved. In its last annual report, *Shaping the Future*, the World Health Organization (WHO) has underscored this crying need, stating that the 'key task of the global community is to close the gap between such contrasting lives' (WHO, 2003).

It is only through this larger, collective responsibility that India will be able to deliver basic health services to all its citizens. The burden of disease that we suffer today is still not so large and unmanageable that any one sector would find it difficult to address. Nevertheless, be it the government, the voluntary sector, or inspired individuals, the effort has to be a combined one. In fact, experiences in managing the health needs of people over the last five decades and more have shown that this partnership is perhaps the best way out. The health sector needs a visionary approach to be able to sort out the mess it is in today. But then is it really in a mess? Several health professionals, government officials, non-government organizations and individuals would perhaps agree, but a quick analysis of the facts reveals that things are not so dismal after all. There are islands of effort—successful community-level programmes and government projects; efficient, well-run hospitals and clinics; inspired individuals working to deliver strong and effective health services—but the larger picture is, at the cost of sounding pessimistic, dismal. The *Human Development Report (HDR) 2003* has highlighted the real challenge for India: if it weren't for the country's low health indices, it would have been higher on the world chart of Human Development Indices. The inadequacy of the health sector, rampant malnutrition and high infant mortality are pressure points on the overall progress of our nation today.

In India, every problem is magnified owing to its large population of a billion plus. So it is with disease burden and ill health. While there are many health indices that reveal progress and a general betterment in the delivery of good health to all from the time a modern, democratically elected

Indian government took over the running of the country in 1947, India's disease burden continues to be enormous, much more than in many other developing countries with similar economies, and, of course, significantly higher than that in the developed nations of the world. The most unfortunate aspect of this burden is the fact that a large number of illnesses and compromised health situations that people find themselves in are because of infections that can be prevented simply and effectively. Acute respiratory infections, diarrhoea and cholera, besides tuberculosis and malaria, are major challenges to health in India, and all these are diseases that have proven, preventive techniques. The course that modern medicine worldwide has taken, of offering curative care more efficiently and with much easier accessibility than basic preventive methods, has been accepted in India with a totality that is almost frightening, and the evidence of this is in the figures of morbidity and mortality from these preventable infectious diseases. Meanwhile, some 5.1 million Indians are living with the Human Immunodeficiency Virus (HIV) or full-blown Acquired Immunodeficiency Syndrome (AIDS) (National AIDS Control Organization, 2004), the most recent addition to an already long list of infectious diseases.

Some of the existing infectious diseases are now showing up in multi-drug resistant forms, and this is particularly dangerous in the case of tuberculosis (TB), cholera and malaria. Non-communicable, so-called lifestyle diseases are a large part of the burden too. The incidence of coronary heart disease has grown steadily in the past few decades from about 4 per cent in the 1960s to 10 per cent today (*Manorama Year Book*, 2003) and about 25,000 heart bypass surgeries are performed each year. The statistical analysis of data on heart diseases is a challenge because of inadequate and often inappropriate death certification (Reddy, 1998), and there are only small, localized surveys that provide a glimpse of what the nationwide condition would be like. Reddy reports that coronary heart disease in Delhi in 1962 was 5.5 per cent in the high-income group; the same has gone up to 10.9 per cent now. Hypertension too is a condition seen in 10–20 per cent of all urban Indians, and in 10–12 per cent of rural Indians. Cancer, diabetes, and many such diseases also make significant contributions to the health problems faced on a day-to-day basis.

All health challenges get further magnified in the case of women. In a society—at least in most communities—where women are subjugated and stifled by traditional practices that force them to remain the so-called 'weaker' sex, it is almost an accepted fact that the health vulnerabilities of women are much more than average societal indices. In most states of India, conventional societal norms have created such a situation that even as the country moves through the first decade of the third millennium, women are still searching for a voice. In the case of those who have found it, it is either too weak a voice, or it has been with the support of organizations or individuals working to uplift the condition of women. Death during pregnancy or delivery is still common across the country and women who lose their lives during this most natural of life's processes account for a disturbing quarter of all the world's maternal deaths. According to the Ministry of Health and Family Welfare's (MHFW) *Annual Report, 2002–03*, more than 100,000 women die each year from pregnancy and child-birth related causes—this places the country average of maternal mortality at a high ratio of 407 per 100,000 live births. In some of the developed nations of the world this figure is around 10 per 100,000 and even in neighbouring Sri Lanka, it is around 60 per 100,000 (UNDP, 2002). In India, more than half of these deaths are because of haemorrhage, anaemia and sepsis, and these deaths are preventable if women were to have access to very basic obstetric care. Besides the inadequacy of facilities for safe motherhood, women also carry other disease burdens, a condition made worse by their poorer nutritional status as compared to men, and their limited access to good, healthy food on a continuing basis. Added to this is the fact that unhealthy women adversely impact on the health of their children. While the infant mortality rate has declined steadily over the years, and is now down to 70 per 1000 live babies, those who lose their lives are largely neonatal babies (64 per cent) according to the MHFW. These deaths occur because many of the newborns are low birthweight babies, or are born premature. Children also suffer because of a lack of effective and total coverage by the universal immunization programme.

The burden of mental diseases is also growing and one estimate places the number of people who need mental health care, of some kind or the other, at anywhere between 20 and 30 million (National Human Rights Commission, 1999). This number becomes significant when one considers the kind of social stigma that colours mental disorders of any kind, especially in the conventional communities of India. Even finding the appropriate treatment for mentally challenged people is very difficult for the same reason. Surveys have shown that there are just three psychiatrists available per million population, and one bed per 40,000 people (*India Book of the Year 2002*). It was in the year 2001 that WHO decided to focus on mental health in its annual report; this was also the year when the National Human Rights Commission published an exhaustive report on the state of mental hospitals in the country, and of course, they were found to be in a deplorable condition. Ironically, the same year witnessed the tragedy of an all-consuming fire in a so-called mental asylum in Tamil Nadu that not only killed many unsuspecting patients, but also put the spotlight on the manner in which mentally ill patients were being treated across the country. Did all the activity of the year really help? Has the status of mental health institutions improved significantly since then? Are the mentally sick able to knock on more doors now? These are uncomfortable questions, and no guesses for what the answers might be.

The implementation of suggested reform, upkeep and maintenance of existing infrastructure, continuous inputs into the education of medical professionals, policing of ethical practice, regulation of the spread of doctors across the country—in short, oiling and cleaning the machinery that exists so that it runs to maximum efficiency—are the areas wherein lies the biggest faultline in India's health-care sector, whether public or private. The National Health Policy (NHP) of 2002—coming almost two decades after the previous one of 1983—can boast of being an exceptionally forward-looking document with candid admittance of drawbacks in the system: missed goals and targets, and problems that plague the sector. Ideally, such a truthful policy should be able to revolutionize the way in which health care is handed out to ordinary citizens. It should be able to usher in the much-needed reform without trouble because, after all, once the government sets goals for itself there are few who would stand in the way of its achieving these goals. But will that happen in the next five, ten, fifteen years? Although there will be some success, larger reform is going to be extremely difficult. But in a country where there are formal systems to administer health care to every citizen, huge infrastructural networks of hospitals, clinics, primary health-care centres and dispensaries, and significant developments in government policy, it is important to understand why it is so difficult to achieve health-care reform. The reasons as usual are many, over-population being one of them. Every disease and its impact is magnified simply because of the number of people it is likely to affect. Nutrition and health care is a constant worry not just for the people but also for the government, and for many who live in poverty, attaining the purchasing power to actually buy the grain that is filling India's granaries is a far-off dream. Although over-population may be one of the most important reasons behind the inefficiency in the health sector, there are many others that need to be addressed more effectively.

Managing the existing resources judiciously and allocating adequate funds to the health sector are other important issues that need to be looked at. On an average, public health spending rests at an abysmally low Rs 200 per person per year—so low that it leaves many international experts almost speechless. The health budget is an enormous challenge in India and without some revolutionary reform in the way health programmes are budgeted and provided for financially, progress in the health sector in India is going to remain as snail-paced and half-baked as it has been in the past few decades. While aggregate expenditure on health is 5.2 per cent of the gross domestic product (GDP), investment in public health has actually slipped from 1.3 per cent in 1990 to 0.9 per cent in 1999 of the GDP. According to the MHFW, the percentage of the total central budget that is allocated for health remained almost stagnant through the 1990s, at 1.3 per cent, and declined in the states from 7 per cent to 5.5 per cent. The NHP of 2002 recognizes the fact that if countrywide health programmes overall were to get a fillip, there would be a need for 'the injection of substantial resources into the health sector from the Central Budget'. That the government recognizes this urgent need is cause for optimism.

There is also the pressing problem of human resources: not in actual numbers of doctors, but in the kind of motivation and codes of ethical practice that exist in the medical profession today. While the large population has always been a challenge to the available number of doctors and health-care providers, there is also a disturbing lack of motivation that has to be addressed. Over the years, medical professionals—who were outside the purview of any consumer protection act or legal redressal system till less than a decade ago—have had a free run in India, regardless of the ultimate result of their practices, surgical procedures or treatment options. Pushed by the totally unregulated and businesslike growth of the private sector health-care system, the erosion of medical ethics stands complete and, till very recently, remained unchallenged. It is only now that patients who have been wronged have a real voice in the courts, can expect monetary settlements—however small and inadequate—for the traumatic losses that they suffer at the hands of unethical medical practitioners, and even hope for justice from the courts of law in terms of blacklisting of doctors or unethical medical institutions.

This change has proved to be very costly for the ordinary person who is also made to feel guilty for having violated the nobility of the doctor–patient relationship. There have been very long and lonely battles, causing incalculable trauma, anguish and pain, and sometimes the loss of lives of dear ones. And even after claims of many patients have been settled, it is still very difficult to pick a fight with the doctor who, for most average Indians, is still very close to God, and God is not to be displeased or questioned. To this day, a large number of doctors do not like to be asked any questions about their choice of treatment, accuracy of their diagnosis or options available to the patient. Among individuals, who have decided to fight for their right to good health by taking on errant doctors or medical institutions, there are many who have faced outright threats to scuttle their endeavours. And yet, strong and proactive legal interventions from the courts, motivated individuals and consumer action groups and a core of medical professionals who believe in the strongest medical ethics are changing this sad situation into one where there is hope and justice.

The other troubling aspect of human resource involved in providing health care is the acute shortage of doctors willing to serve, at least limited terms, in rural and less-privileged urban areas. This scarcity has been felt over the years and it will not be wrong to say that it has been a major factor in the disease burden being shouldered by people who live in these areas. The NHP of 2002 recognizes the need for what it calls 'policy initiatives' to change this scenario—but how exactly the government plans to get medical professionals to go to a place where they are perhaps needed the most is not clear, and this may prove tougher than has been envisaged by politicians and bureaucrats.

In fact, the strong political vision and will, needed to keep a nation's health system intact, have been grossly inadequate in the past few decades. While environmental reform has received considerable attention from governments, health has always been a low priority, and this indifference has been brought to light in the last few years. In just two years, over 2002–03, the Bharatiya Janata Party-led coalition government saw three health ministers run this all-important ministry—Dr C.P. Thakur, Mr Shatrughan Sinha, and Ms Sushma Swaraj. With the change in government, Dr A. Ramadoss took charge of the health ministry in June 2004. While Thakur was at least a medical doctor and had a good grasp of the health scenario and its problems (a skill that is perhaps reflected in some measure in the strong NHP of 2002 released during his tenure), Mr Sinha brought no special talent to a difficult job, that of running the MHFW in a country where the burden of disease is high and the challenges of administering the public health infrastructure are daunting to even the most skilled person on the job. Sinha was criticized for his casual and indifferent approach to the job at hand, but it is important to ask tough questions to the central command of the party that put him in the wrong place. Ms Swaraj rekindled hope in the hearts of many health workers and organizations simply because of her political track record in handling other ministries, but some irrational interventions by her ministry in basic prevention programmes, such as the use of condoms to ward off HIV infection, were not taken very lightly. At a time when the larger Indian community was beginning to come out of the shadows to use condoms freely, recognizing the importance of this simple device in practising safe sex and therefore as a very basic protection from AIDS, this kind of policy reversal could create a heavy negative impact that may prove difficult to rectify. Political parties and senior political leaders, at their individual levels, will have to show much more interest in the health-care sector and in its many trials and tribulations for any real and tangible reform to set in. In current analysis, pre-election party manifestos make disturbingly minimal reference to health-related issues.

Some of India's improving health indices have been celebrated in the past few years, but the clouds return when comparisons are drawn, and these could be comparisons with other countries anywhere in the world, or between different states and union territories within India, or even between city and village dwellers in India. The indices of success then suddenly pale and the faultlines begin to show once more. In the global scenario, standard health indices for India still compare poorly with world averages, and are unable to stand comparison even with much smaller countries like Sri Lanka where health has always been a priority for human development. Within India too, there are so many variations in the progress of health of the people that the national averages very often seem far removed from reality. If there are 267 mothers who lose their lives for every 100,000 births in urban areas, the figure is a disturbingly high 619 in rural areas. Again, in the state of Uttar Pradesh, maternal mortality ratios are as high as 707 in 100,000 births, against only 29 in Gujarat. Infant mortality is 89 for every 1000 live births in Meghalaya, but only 16.3 in Kerala. If this is inequity, this is also an inability to try and replicate successful model programmes where they could have made a difference to the lives of ordinary people. Many reasons have been put forth over the years as to why a health or education programme that works in Kerala or Goa cannot be transported to a setting in Uttar Pradesh or Bihar, but none of them are really convincing or compelling enough. Somewhere, again, the needle on the dial swings to political effort, mobilization and motivation. If government delegations can go to the United Kingdom or the United States of America on state-sponsored visits to study their transport systems and sewage lines, surely programmes from India's progressive states can become workable in the states where they are really needed.

Of course, it means a lot of work. But if the country's tourism industry can, by the simple approach of creating attractive spaces for the easy spirit, put together with such far-sighted diligence 'total health' programmes that cost the earth but bring in precious foreign exchange, then the less glamorous but more pressing needs of millions in India can also be met: indeed they must be met! Is there a choice? Can we continue to ignore the needless deaths of children from diseases that a simple, accessible vaccine could have prevented? Can we truly say we have tried our best to wipe out the pointless deaths of mothers as they deliver babies they have nursed in their wombs for nine long months? Are we doing whatever can be done to reduce the growing burden of heart disease? Honestly, the answer is no to all these and more questions we might wish to ask about meeting the health-care needs of our people. But, will these dark clouds not blow away? True, the leaden weight of varied and diverse diseases and disorders is part of India's reality, and also the world's, but it is not a challenge that cannot be overcome. In fact, there has been some success in tackling these challenges and trying to find solutions to them so as to make things better. As always, there is reason for optimism and all of it is based on true stories of reform, of positive impact, of real and tangible improvement in the health and well-being of people. There are strong beacons of light showing the way ahead. These could be individuals fired with the inspiration to do something to better people's lives; these could also be groups and organizations, larger charitable institutions, and very often, the government. The anti-tobacco and anti-cigarette smoking campaigns have taken root across various states with the ban on smoking in public places, fines for violators, abolition of the sale of tobacco products to non-adults, and with the banning of advertisements of tobacco products on television (*India Book of the Year 2002*). Sex selection through prenatal testing of unborn foetuses has also been banned and the Supreme Court has laid emphasis on the need for a more proactive role by the centre and state governments in ensuring the effectiveness of the ban.

The *NHP, 2002*, admitting to the increasingly significant role the private sector is now playing in handing out health to people, says:

> With the increasing role of private health care, the implementation of statutory regulation, and the monitoring of minimum standards of diagnostic centres/medical institutions become imperative. The Policy will address issues regarding the establishment of a comprehensive information system, and based on that the establishment of a regulatory mechanism to ensure the maintaining of adequate standards by diagnostic centres/medical institutions, as well as the proper conduct of clinical practice and delivery of medical services.

The same logic has also been extended to the non-governmental sector. The *NHP, 2002* says:

> Currently, non-governmental service providers are treating a large number of patients at the primary level for major diseases. However, the treatment regimens followed are diverse and not scientifically optimal, leading to an increase in the incidence of drug resistance. The policy will address itself to recommending arrangements which will eliminate the risks arising from inappropriate treatment.

Strong government policy—and more importantly, implementation of that policy—together with far-reaching, efficient non-governmental efforts, and inspired individuals dedicated to reform, can definitely help improve the health-care scene in India. There is no way but to build partnerships and involve the community that needs to be served, and also no way but to take small-scale, local approaches to solving

India's health problems. The good news is that many of these localized, micro-community approaches are already working wonders, and just up-scaling them will also be a giant step towards progress. As long as the various people and institutions involved in taking that step realize the urgency of doing so, there is a lot that can be changed in the way India's health-care systems are being administered and in the way health care is being delivered to people. That achieved, it takes little imagination to comprehend that the progress of health status of Indians would be a significant contribution to the overall strength of the country in the global scheme of things.

India's Killers: The Big and the Not-So-Big

The optimism of a relatively few years ago that many of these diseases could easily be brought under control has led to a fatal complacency among the international community. This complacency is now costing millions of lives—lives that we have the knowledge and the means to save, yet we are allowing to trickle through our fingers.

—Dr Hiroshi Nakajima, former Director General, World Health Organization (WHO), 1996

Dr Anita Nair* is a woman who breathes and belongs in the great Indian city. She is the perfect example of a successful career woman—a good education, fulfilling career experience and a life that wants for nothing. The 'Dr' that she can proudly prefix to her name has always made her heart swell, for, behind it lie many years of university education. She is forever busy, running against each twenty-four-hour day, packing in as much as she can between sunrise and sunset, and often filling the remaining hours stretching her healthy body to its limits between home and work. Her other constant

---

* The names of some people have been changed to protect their privacy.

source of joy is the good health she has always maintained. It was also one reason for her mother's joy, who derived solace from the fact that her younger daughter's good health would see her through the gruelling routine of her life.

Anita had always enjoyed the spoils of this ability of her body and its remarkable immune system that managed to consistently ward off illness. The thirty-five-year-old journalist living in New Delhi had stray, scant memories of sickness. That is how things were till the end of yet another hard day in August of 1997, when Anita was driving home from work late at night. An uncomfortably warm flush spread through her and she experienced a sudden blurring of her vision. For a brief but awful moment, the headlights from the traffic coming from the opposite direction merged into one blinding wall of brightness. Blinking quickly and trying desperately to focus on the shiny fender of the vehicle just ahead of her, Anita felt a great surge of exhaustion, almost as if her body would collapse. As she drove, Anita tried to recall if something had gone wrong that day, and she realized that she had perhaps been running a fever throughout the day. Now that she thought about it, she had constantly ignored her body signals. She had felt what her sister's husband, who was also their family doctor, would have called a malaise: a general feeling of listlessness and lack of well-being.

'Some nasty virus, I guess,' Anita spoke to herself, already worrying about her deadline the next day. When her husband answered the doorbell, he looked aghast. 'What's up, Ani?' he asked, very anxious, which is when Anita realized that she must be looking awful. 'I think I've been running a fever all day; why, do I look that bad?' Anita asked. 'You just need to be in bed,' said her husband. She looked ready to collapse. Pumped with anti-pyretics, Anita felt better as the night wore on, and by the next morning the fever had gone. It returned, however, but so many days later that Anita did not even connect it with the earlier episode. A sweaty Delhi August gave way to a slightly better September. The fever often recurred, but it was so low-grade that neither Anita nor her husband, or anybody else in the family for that matter, felt that she needed to do anything about it, other than popping the usual anti-pyretic. Soon, Anita began to notice her very low energy levels. Mundane tasks seemed impossible and it took all her strength just to go through a regular day.

Amazingly, neither Anita nor anybody else in her circle of family and friends saw anything amiss and two of Anita's favourite months—October and November—passed with the otherwise energetic woman unable to do anything more than what she had to for subsistence. But somehow, again, nobody noticed the subtle fading of her otherwise undying spunk. As winter came on, Anita developed a nagging cough that bothered her so much that she couldn't even conduct a proper conversation on the phone, not something a journalist could ever be happy about! She must have downed a few litres of cough syrup, but to no avail. Her brother-in-law too dismissed it as a regular winter cough and nobody felt the need for any advanced tests to nail the cough and find a reason for Anita's listlessness. And, when the cough suddenly disappeared after two weeks, everybody happily attributed it to a short warm spell in January. But the fatigue had increased and as the months wore on, Anita's family began commenting on her loss of weight. Very happy that her exercises and diet had finally worked, she gave little thought to the fact that her weight had actually dropped too drastically. Meanwhile, the cough also came back, and by April, she had learnt to live with it and with a nagging pain along her left shoulder. There was one enormous source of happiness though: she was now fitting into jeans she had worn before her daughter was born!

Finally one morning in May 1998, just after they had celebrated her daughter's sixth birthday, Anita wondered why she didn't feel happy when everybody at the party commented on how much slimmer she looked from the last time they had seen her. As she brushed her teeth, she noticed a large lump at the curve, where her neck bone joined the shoulder. Again, giving it little thought, she carelessly rubbed a pain-relief balm over it, connecting the shoulder pain with this swelling. But two days later, when she explained all this to a close friend who worked as a radiologist in Delhi's Indraprastha Apollo Hospital, he didn't like the sound of what she described. 'Come over, and let me have a look,' he said, trying to sound as casual and noncommittal as possible. But knowing him as well as she did, Anita was quick to catch something in his voice, something that went straight to her heart, and for the first time in months she was really worried.

But the phone call had been worth it. At last, Anita was in good hands. As soon as her doctor friend saw the lump, his face fell. Anita, cursing herself silently for having ignored her illness over the months, thought it must be cancer. She felt strangely detached, as though she was waiting to hear about somebody else's illness, not her own. Before the afternoon wore out they had gone through a test called Fine Needle Aspiration Cytology (FNAC), and while the news was bad, it wasn't cancer. Tuberculosis (TB) was to be her cross to bear. 'It could have been much worse, right?' said her friend, giving her a warm hug. Sure it could have been awful; after all, TB was curable, right? But the relief was only half-hearted. 'How come I have TB?' Anita wanted to shout in the cool, quiet, sterile hospital corridor, and her husband, knowing how she felt, said in his quiet way: 'You're going to be fine'.

The real reason why she was so upset was because Anita knew too much about the disease for comfort. Well-read and highly educated, she knew what she was down with—a terrible and debilitating disease that could prove fatal if one was not careful with the medication. For her mother and mother-in-law the news was totally devastating simply because in their day nobody survived TB. Yet, it was something else that secretly pained everybody—that they had waited ten long months before getting Anita's illness diagnosed, and that it took a big and visible lump to goad them into action. And if this was the response in an educated family, it is scary to think what it must be like in the homes of millions of less-fortunate people. Well, at least they acted, and that they did became the difference between life and death for Anita.

The Deadly Germ within Us

Thousands of Indians are not half as lucky as Anita. Just as it was with her, all these people live with nagging coughs, low fevers that linger for months, and slow-but-steady weight loss. Never do they stop to check what really ails them. Coughs are so commonplace, as are fevers and fatigue, that for many Indians who are busy just living their lives and trying to earn enough to get by, the thought of visiting a doctor doesn't even cross their minds. And this must be the plight of several people because, according to *Annual Report, 2002–03*, published by the Ministry of Health and Family Welfare (MHFW), in India one person succumbs to TB every minute leading to 450,000–500,000 people dying each year of TB. With at least 15 million active TB cases to which 2.2 million are added every year, India accounts for nearly a third of the world's total TB patients. It is now no longer a disease brought on by poverty, squalor or malnutrition, and there are countless men and women like Anita who are battling against TB. This disease is the biggest killer in Southeast Asia, where 95 per cent of all TB cases are found across five countries: India, Bangladesh, Myanmar, Thailand and Indonesia. Unofficially, most people who die of AIDS actually die because of TB. More than half, almost 80 per cent, of all AIDS cases diagnosed in India are people suffering from TB as well (WHO, 1998).

TB, caused by the bacterium *Mycobacterium tuberculosis*, lives within many of us in what some might call a friendly relationship. It is still not clear as to what really brings on a full-blown infection, except, of course, in the case of people exposed to the infectious disease in some way, but it is clearly a response to a compromised immune system. And once the bacterium shows up, it becomes a contagion deeply debilitating in its overall impact. This resilient germ that has made such a strong base for itself inside the bodies of so many people can completely ruin the lungs, clog the lymph nodes (that is what Anita's shoulder lump was), or colonize the bones. Anita always believed the germ within her came up for air because of her exaggerated attempts at dieting to lose weight. 'I was compromising so much on my food, maybe the germ got the better of my immune system,' she says. Such is the mystery of disease and death that the real reason for the bacillus winning the battle against Anita's antibodies may never be revealed. This is the case with one of the most serious health problems in India, TB, but much the same mystery often underlies the history of communicable diseases that have continued to confound human knowledge and the advancement of science. The TB bacillus is an opportunistic infection, quickly turning from a harmless bodily presence into a monster that can conquer and devour one's natural immune response if the right amount of drugs to beat the bacterium are not taken. Anita was fortunate because her specific ailment turned out to be of the non-infectious kind, so she was able to continue living the way she had before she was diagnosed. Yet, she kept her disease a well-guarded secret. That TB is contagious in its most conventional form makes it difficult for many ordinary people to accept a person with active TB into their daily circle of friends or family. For Anita too there was more comfort in keeping the news of her illness a secret, anathema to her extrovert and forward-looking personality. She took no comfort in the fact that today TB is a disease that is spreading across societal lines and social boundaries. Earlier considered a disease that people from less economically privileged classes suffered from, it has of late got itself a white-collar tag. White-collar TB is no longer snazzy jargon, but harsh reality. Anita is a typical example of the fact that TB can strike the well-fed, well-looked-after person as well. In a survey of AIDS-related TB cases in Mumbai, the AIDS Research and Control Centre (ARCON) of the Brihanmumbai Municipal Corporation found that the percentage of people from the middle and upper classes (earning over Rs 12,000 a month) suffering from the disease had risen from 12 per cent in 1994 to 48 per cent in 1996 (Abreu and Menon, 1997).

Fortunately, TB can be cured, but there is a caveat to this. The drug regimen is tough and long, and even the slightest slip-up in the consumption of these strong drugs can cause a relapse. After her initial diagnosis, Anita contacted a senior specialist at the All India Institute of Medical Sciences (AIIMS) in New Delhi. Confirming the diagnosis after a thorough examination, the doctor told Anita: 'You should stop thinking of yourself as an unusual case. You would be surprised if I tell you how many people I am treating.' While this brought some solace to Anita, she was also intimidated by what he went on to say. He explained the drug regimen to her, and told her not to miss out on a single dose. 'You will soon be cured,' he said, 'but defaulting on this regimen can bring the germ back in its drug-resistant form. So, don't try it.' At first she resented his attitude, but then realized how seriously he meant what he was saying. Death from ordinary TB comes only to patients who default on the drug regimen. It was Anita's realization and acceptance of this fact that went on to make the all-important difference between life and death in the months to come. Even short-term chemotherapy takes six to nine months. Anita stuck to it knowing her life depended on it, consuming four strong drugs at different times of the day for two months, and then two drugs for the rest of the course of treatment.

But there was something else she was totally unprepared for. While Anita often thought in her most private moments about dying of the disease, the real killing came each day: the daily trauma of deep-set fatigue, the chronic bouts of coughing, an almost undetectable fever, a lack of interest in food, and the total lack of interest in things that had always excited her. Losing 5 kg was perhaps the least traumatic and most visual of the impact that this terrible infection was having on her; the others were the real scars that it left on Anita. She was right, the TB bacillus can kill a person in many different ways. And as she found, it is a disease with the capacity to really devastate people's normal lives and cause a great deal of morbidity. That is why health experts calculate the real burden of TB not as loss of life, but as a daily disability that can affect work, health and happiness. Disability Adjusted Life Years (DALY) is a measure that combines the burden suffered from premature death with that of living with a disability. This is considered to be an established way of expressing the morbidity of TB. The respiratory discomfort, combined with persistent low-grade fever and what seems like unconquerable fatigue affect a person's ability to think and function properly, leaving a serious impact on his or her natural working capacity. According to the Tuberculosis Research Centre in Chennai, total life years lost due to the sickness that TB brings stands at 62.8 lakh DALYs for men and 45.6 lakh DALYs for women (Prabhakar and Narayanan, 1996).

Now, five safe years have passed and Anita has shown no signs of relapse. A few months into the drug therapy, her lump vanished, the cough disappeared, and the weight she had lost came back. 'That's the only sad part,' she says jokingly now, but after all that she went through, the extra weight is something she will gladly carry forever. On an average, TB patients find it difficult to stick by the drug regimen. The problem is that the drugs show their effect very quickly and the otherwise run-down patient begins to feel better. He/she becomes lax, forgetting to take the drugs regularly, and becomes a defaulter. When people die of TB, they die because they stop taking the drugs, bored with the strict and long regimen, satisfied with feeling better very quickly. What these defaulters do not realize is that besides being unable to cure themselves of a disease that can be fatal, they also allow the germ within them to learn to live with the antibiotics that are actually meant to kill it, because they don't allow the full dosage required to overpower the germ to enter their system. When a patient halts the drug regimen prematurely, the bacillus still within slowly learns to survive against the baseline concentration of the antibiotics that would kill the bacillus in full force. This, happening over many years and in millions of people across the world, has created little Frankensteins of the original bacterium, resistant to traditional drugs. Multi-drug resistant TB (MDR TB) requires stronger and more expensive drugs, whose curative capacity is not certain, and which can have strong adverse effects. Drug regimens for MDR TB can cost up to Rs 2.5 lakh for the complete course while ordinary TB can be treated for a maximum of Rs 5000 (Abreu and Menon, 1997). Some years ago, when doctors at the Armed Forces Medical College in Pune decided to look carefully into the spread of drug-resistant TB, they picked 4011 patients from the armed forces. While 40.4 per cent soldiers showed a TB-positive culture, resistance to any single drug was seen in 12.5 per cent, and 4.7 per cent of the soldiers were resistant to two drugs. This was a study done between April 1992 and December 1995. Chances are that this number has gone up many times. MDR TB is growing in urban areas and could be anywhere between 3 and 6 per cent in the community at large. At King Edward Memorial (KEM) College, Mumbai, MDR TB has been showing an alarming increase, from 7321 cases in 1994 to 14,448 in 1996 (Abreu and Menon, 1997). At New Delhi's AIIMS too, microbiologists have found 63 per cent of sputum samples showing drug-resistant bacteria.

The only way to ensure a reduction in this burden is to have systems in place that can monitor drug regimens. Unlike Anita, there are millions of Indians who require assistance in following this long and strenuous treatment. They lack the awareness, empowerment or luxury to stick to the routine. This one facet of TB treatment was the biggest drawback of the National Tuberculosis Control Programme—it had not managed to work out a simple door-to-door monitoring system for the management of this regimen. Meanwhile, the WHO had popularized Directly Observed Short-term Treatment or DOTS for TB, in which a health worker physically stands and watches a TB patient as he or she takes the drugs. Around the time that Anita was battling against

TB, the Indian government launched what it calls the Revised National TB Control Programme (RNTCP), based on DOTS, in 1997. According to the government, 500 million Indians have since been covered under the programme (*Annual Report, 2002–03*), and this has apparently shown treatment success rates of 84 per cent: thrice the 25 per cent success rate that was achieved in the earlier programme. Since the RNTCP took over, a little less than 5 per cent of patients testing positive in the smear test have died; the burden of mortality was 29 per cent in the earlier programme. 'The RNTCP has saved more than 230,000 lives and prevented more than 26,00,000 TB infections,' says the *Annual Report, 2002–03*.

But TB remains one of India's biggest killers. It is indeed surprising that the first effective programme is only a few years old. Also, there are reports that often TB patients are sent back from the hospital with an ordinary cough mixture. Few Indians even know that the only cure for TB is to go through the prescribed drug regimen without defaulting. Even fewer people are aware that considering how infectious TB can be, a cured patient also does society a good turn. Anita was surprised when her doctor told her that by curing herself, she has also shouldered her social responsibility by removing the bacterium from yet another niche it had found for itself— her body. As far as TB goes, some of the unwarranted complacency has also come from the Bacillus Calmette-Guerin (BCG) vaccine that is administered in infancy. Most people believe that this vaccine will protect the vaccinated against the disease. But that is not so. The vaccine simply provides protection in childhood against miliary TB. This is not to say that protection against this form of TB is not necessary. It is in itself a great enough contribution to public health, considering the fatal effects TB can have in childhood. It is only that ordinary people need to be informed about this, and they should be clearly told that the neonatal BCG vaccination will in no way guarantee a TB-free adulthood (For further information see Box: The BCG Conundrum, pp. 37–38). TB brought on by HIV infection also complicates the scenario immensely, causing more deaths and morbidity. Way back in 1992, scientists at the Department of Microbiology in Pune surveyed this dual infection and found 1.18 per cent of all TB patients to be HIV positive. The same figure had grown to 4.43 per cent in 1999. With all these new dimensions, this old scourge is still one of India's prime health challenges. Amazingly similar is the case of a large number of vector-borne diseases, where bacteria and viruses carried by insects cause disease and death.

The Mosquitoes Are Back

Rohan Kumar* was the regular boy-next-door. He had lots of friends, they played basketball together, watched movies, went jogging and cycling. He was his parents' only child, went to school in Delhi and led the usual, fun-filled life of a teenager. Then one day something happened to change this handsome, young boy's life forever (Menon, 1996). A mosquito bit him. Scores of mosquitoes bite countless people each day and we don't give it a second thought, do we? But this mosquito was different—*Aedes aegyptii*, city-bred, black and white striped, and carrier of the infamous dengue virus. Rohan was admitted to a large private hospital in Delhi. As Rohan's parents watched over him anxiously, his body began fighting the virus with antibodies. But soon, another strain of the virus put a stop to this improvement and this time, the boy's body temperature shot up to a 105°F, strained by the infection. The germ was on a mission, breaking down his vital platelet cells which would in normal course help his blood to clot. In that young, ravaged body, the blood began to thin out abnormally, oozing out through the nose and the mouth. His blood pressure plummeted and he sank into a coma that doctors call the dengue shock syndrome. At the end of two weeks and what must have been a terribly anguished time, Rohan gave up the struggle. To think that a robust boy poised for life should be lost to the world because of a mosquito bite is so sad and traumatic that it makes one wonder what life is really all about.

More than 500 people perished in this epidemic that shook Delhi out of complacency in 1996—a statistic made painfully significant by the fact that it was totally and simply avoidable. It was dengue and its wilder form, dengue haemorrhagic fever, that caused the painful resurgence of an epidemic and sent shock waves throughout the capital because they killed people from all classes of society, with no regard for economic strength or affluent lifestyle. The dengue mosquito is a dangerous cousin of the more common one that causes malaria. There is a set of four dengue viruses that causes dengue and dengue haemorrhagic fever, two closely-related conditions. This is a disease considered by public health experts as among the most dangerous to humans, especially as a major emerging tropical viral disease that can quickly transport a person from total well-being to death. Senior virologists had even predicted the 1996 outbreak and feel terribly saddened that no action was ever taken in spite of these predictions. Dengue affects more than 100 countries across the world and there are some 20 million people who fall sick each year, with 500,000 in need of hospitalization (WHO, 1996). Yet, it must be said that the quick deaths that Delhi's dengue epidemic caused across socio-economic borders did make health authorities sit up, for a while at least. Health workers went about fumigating the city, and conducting regular checks on water coolers in homes and offices. Proactivity ruled. That is more than one can say for the TB bacillus which, over the many centuries that it has been around, has lulled the medical and health community into a resigned, let's-live-with-it kind of attitude. The fact is there: it is no longer a great shock to contract the disease and it can—albeit with great effort—be cured. The dengue virus has none of the excuses that *M. tuberculosis* gets away with. It does not reside within us, nor is it airborne. Yet, in connivance with the diehard mosquito, it is spreading ill health, even death, simply because of inefficient community health programmes. A total indifference and nonchalance on part of the general community towards keeping our surroundings clean has further encouraged such epidemics. Major cities in India have seen a spurt in the mosquito population over the past few years. Nothing seems to work against them. While some of us simply feel helpless and frustrated, for others, it is much more than just frustration. For Rohan's family, the seemingly insignificant mosquito today stands for a vacuous sadness that never seems to go away.

If this is not shame enough on the country's public health infrastructure, what is? Today, Rohan's parents may have tried to move on and bear their anguish, but that is more than one can say for the government and the country's health infrastructure. After the first few years since the 1996 outbreak in the capital, it is business as usual. Diligent health workers' visits to check for breeding mosquito population have stopped. As documented in the *Annual Report, 2002–03*, the number of reported dengue cases across the country was 1177 in 1997, and with stringent measures taken largely because of the 1996 epidemic, this figure fell to 707 in 1998, rose to 3278 in 2001 and was 748 up to October 2002. In other words, if the government and individuals decide, they can easily control the mosquito population. But a general lack of civic sense among the average Indian population and a lack of concern among government officials have aided and abetted a post-DDT era mosquito menace to grow beyond all calculation. While dengue is still less frequent, malaria refuses to go away. During the past few years, its deadlier version, falciparum malaria (cerebral malaria, caused by *Plasmodium falciparum*; ordinary malaria is caused by *P. vivax*) has been the cause of several deaths, specially in parts of Rajasthan. Moreover, *P. falciparum* has changed its form so often and mutated with such regularity that it is becoming resistant to mainline drugs. More virulent than its cousin *P. vivax*, this strain of the germ causes death in most cases.

Reports have shown that in the district of Bharatpur alone, the total cases of cerebral malaria shot up fourfold to almost 16,000 within a single year (1995–96). The government is working through its Enhanced Malaria Control Project to try and bring things under control in Bharatpur. Other areas like Jaipur, Dholpur, Savai Madhopur and Dausa have also reported increases in the number of people coming down with malaria over the years. Earlier only 10–20 per cent of all malaria cases used to be cerebral, but now this figure has gone up to 40 per cent. When civil engineers conceived of and created the Indira Gandhi Canal, people were excited about the prospect of bringing water to an arid zone. Today, experts of communicable diseases explain how this very canal served as the perfect breeding ground for mosquitoes. The canal also caused a total change in the area's ecosystem, transforming the dry, hot countryside to wet and hot—the mosquito's favourite habitat. It is the same story with crowded urban housing where badly maintained overhead tanks create the ambience that the mosquito thrives on.

Rajasthan may be in the news, but it is the northeast that

suffers the real onslaught of this terrible disease year after year. Scientists at the Regional Medical Research Centre (Northeastern Region) of the Indian Council for Medical Research (ICMR) have recently studied the possible risk factors of malaria in the thick rainforests of Arunachal Pradesh (Mohapatra et al., 2001). These are parts of the country where the disease is most concentrated and vengeful. According to the MHFW, the northeastern states contribute between 8 and 11 per cent of the total cases of malaria in the country.

Thus, more than half a century after Independence, and close to four decades since the National Malaria Eradication Programme (NMEP) was first formulated, most urban areas in the country still face the threat of malaria. A growing population and changes in lifestyle have aggravated the situation. For instance, if a few urban families in a city had a single air cooler back in the 1960s, today, each family, cutting across all economic sections of society, has anywhere from one to four coolers in their homes. Consumption of water has gone up; the mountains of garbage too have grown, making matters worse.

The government has finally realized that in the present situation, the incidence of malaria can be minimized but can never be completely eradicated. It has thus renamed its NMEP programme as the National Anti-Malaria Programme (NAMP). This is fine as long as there is a minimization or at least a reduction in the cases of malaria and deaths caused by the disease each year. Although the number of cases of malaria each year has reached a steady plateau (2–3 million cases), it is the death rate that is still high. While in 1976 only 59 people succumbed to malaria, right through the 1990s the figure was closer to 1000, and it was 1015 in 2001 (*Annual Report, 2002–03*). It is perhaps so much mortality, repeated outbreaks of resistant falciparum malaria and epidemics like dengue that have taken with them some of the complacency associated with diseases caused by the mosquito.

Some other diseases that are vector-borne—filariasis, which creates elephantine legs in its sufferers, and Japanese encephalitis—have started to show up in alarming numbers. India alone has an estimated 45 million carriers of filariasis and about 19 million people affected (WHO, 1998a). Kerala in fact has recently reported a high incidence of Japanese encephalitis. Mosquitoes breed in rice fields and with large-scale irrigation patterns, this pesky population can sustain itself all through the year. The waves of fever and drowsiness that characterize Japanese encephalitis must be diagnosed early, otherwise the virus can affect the brain. Blood platelet formation dips alarmingly, and this can cause serious damage.

If mosquitoes have made a powerful re-entry in the post-DDT years, so also have sandflies. When DDT was used expansively in the 1950s and 1960s, killing sandflies was a bonus for the NMEP, or what health workers called the collateral benefit of spraying DDT. But their resurgence, that too in resistant forms, has brought kala azar—the often-fatal disease in India's semi-rural areas—back. Confined to east and northeast India, kala azar is caused by a tiny pathogen called *Leishmania donovani*, which brings with it irregular spells of fever, weight loss, a swollen liver and spleen, and anaemia. Visceral leishmaniasis, as kala azar is also called, came back renewed and strengthened in the late 1970s; it can kill each person it infects if he or she is untreated. In 1977, there were at least 4000 deaths in Bihar alone (Bhaduri, 1996).

Viral Load: HIV/AIDS and Much Else

In deadly harmony, old diseases and new are adding to the health challenges that India faces. HIV/AIDS is the king of communicable diseases, having first shown up just two decades ago, but causing so much suffering that everybody is worrying about it now. Not only has it made its way from affecting only high-risk groups in a society that is extremely caste conscious, it has also changed societal balances and relationships. In India, HIV has crossed borders. Government estimates place the number of infected people at 5.1 million (National AIDS Control Organization, 2004). More than 2000 people have died since the first AIDS case was detected in Tamil Nadu in 1986. Today, AIDS is no longer a terrible illness you hear about as affecting the lives of sex workers, truck drivers or drug addicts, but is the image of a husband and wife from an ordinary, middle-class family infected, with nowhere to go. It is a chronic viral infection that refuses to go away, and the new line of drugs is expensive, beyond the reach of many ordinary Indians, which is perhaps why health workers and doctors believe that the only real way out is to closely monitor the population and work hard towards teaching the adolescent population about the disease. AIDS in India is accepted as a big challenge, but there is a number-game being played around it. There are voluntary organizations like the Joint Action Council, Kannur (JACK) that question government statistics on the number of HIV positive people, raising doubts about the figures. On the whole it is evident that whatever be the numbers, there is a pressing need to clarify the controversy and at least have a working estimate of the actual burden of disease from this dangerous viral infection. Considering the stigma associated with it, reportage of cases is a problem and may continue to remain so. Today the spotlight is on AIDS owing to its wide reach as an infection and because there is no cure for it at present.

That is not something one can say for jaundice and viral hepatitis. These virulent and viral infections affect the liver, a major hub of all biological activities in the body. Hepatitis spreads the same way AIDS does, but few people understand how serious the infection can be. The Hepatitis C virus is considered much more resilient than HIV. According to WHO, more than a third of the world's population is infected with the Hepatitis B virus (HBV). In the southeast Asian region alone there are more than 80 million carriers of the virus. When it spreads, estimates are that one in every four infected babies will die of liver cancer or cirrhosis of the liver. The ICMR attributes 1 per cent of all adult deaths in India to HBV (Menon, 1997a). It is the fifth largest killer of people in India in the 14–45 age group, and lives in 3–5 per cent of the total population.

No wonder, Urmila Sehgal considers herself a fortunate woman (Menon, 1997a). Sehgal, a teacher and mother of two children, developed a persistent fever some years ago and, fighting fatigue, tried to live with what she thought was pure inconvenience for some time. But a nose-bleed made her rush to the hospital. Within weeks she became bloated with unspent fluids and a liver-function test showed that the all-important organ had stopped functioning. If Sehgal recovered, it was for two simple reasons. One, she could afford the almost 'magic' drug Interferon with the help of her extended family. Few Indians can afford this drug. Sehgal, for instance, spent about Rs 900 each day and took the injections for a month. Second, Sehgal was lucky that she responded to the drug; not all patients do.

The Small Irritants

These are only a few of the hiccups in treating and tackling infectious diseases. The complexity of the issue in India is that apart from these major infections there are also the commonplace ones to which people give scant attention but which cause large-scale deaths as well. Acute respiratory infections (ARIs) and diarrhoeal disorders kill more people than AIDS, malaria and TB put together. Two-thirds of the children from birth to the tender age of 5 years die of ARIs and diarrhoeal diseases. A study conducted by the Department of Paediatrics at IGM Hospital, Agartala, shows that in Tripura's urban areas (west Tripura district) the monthly incidence of ARIs is 23 per cent and 16 of every 1000 children has pneumonia (Deb, 1998). Diarrhoea, so easily controlled by oral rehydration therapy, causes 18 per cent of all deaths from communicable diseases in the southeast Asian region, and communicable diseases alone are responsible for at least 38 per cent of all deaths. Diarrhoea, health workers always complain, is not even on the horizon as a disease, leave alone reporting or tackling it. Public health experts often feel that we should concentrate on eliminating the disease burden of some of these diseases which can be easily tackled with simple interventional methods.

There is also a high incidence of rabies in India—simply because we prefer not to manage our garbage in a healthy way—and it is adversely affecting people's health and lifespan. Many believe that keeping the environment clean is too simplistic a way of looking at the problem, but like it or not, it is one of the important reasons why rabies is common across the country today. More than 80 per cent of all people who die of rabies in the world are in the southeast Asian region and in India, every year, at least 30,000 people are affected. If only we could contain the population of stray dogs, this disease that can be fatal could be contained to a great extent. Along with rabies, what makes matters really dismal are the daily killers, like cholera and gastroenteritis. Even today, anywhere between 2000 to 10,000 people die of cholera in

India. While cholera always seems distant to the urban elite, caused as it is by a water-borne bacterium, there are no impenetrable barriers here. Then there are the new entrants, like the new strain of cholera caused by Vibrio cholerae 0139. It is less than a decade old and was discovered in India and Bangladesh, but it has fortunately not shown up since 1994 (WHO, 1998a).

From the Shadows

When the plague resurfaced in Beed, Maharashtra and in Surat, Gujarat, after a dormancy of twenty-seven years, the disease threw the country's health infrastructure into a real tizzy and cost India US$ 1.5 billion. Active medical physicians found they had nothing other than historical knowledge about the disease. In fact, after the episode, there were serious discussions about re-introducing plague as a chapter in the section on communicable diseases in the country's medical college curriculums. Plague resurfaced in India's diamond city, which produces some of the country's most expensive jewellery, where day-to-day hygiene on the streets of the city was abysmal. And, as the commissioner of Surat then discovered, the city had simply been ignoring the very basics of health and public hygiene. Bubonic plague resurfaced in a small pocket of Himachal Pradesh in 2002, but the government was able to contain the infection rapidly.

It is said that yellow fever, currently a threat in Africa, may not take long in reaching India. Virologists and doctors in India worry about this fever because the conditions exist for its transmission. The Chikgunya virus lurks in the shadows. It was last recorded in 1973 and cannot be written off, and is known to hit urban and semi-urban areas (Menon, 1996). In 1994, antibodies to the infection that causes Rift Valley fever, otherwise long gone from India, were found among sheep in Rajasthan. The Chandipura virus, first found in patients during a dengue epidemic in Nagpur back in the 1960s, may well be around. Since then, it has also been found in sandflies in Maharashtra. Then there are the Ganjam Virus, Buffalo Pox, and West Nile Fever: the list is endless. Hidden from human vision or research, new germs are constantly evolving, others waiting, forgotten, in the wings. Kyasanur Forest Disease in the Malnad area of Karnataka is another example of how intrusive activities by human society take their toll. So, whether it is a canal in a dry region—which allowed malaria to grow unchecked in Rajasthan—or a lopped forest, or a dam with huge water reservoirs, human activities could aid the emergence of hitherto unknown viruses and bacteria. Meanwhile, as unknown germs emerge, the familiar ones mutate. The conjunctivitis virus is one that is rapidly evolving, and so is the virus that causes diarrhoea. The evolution time span has shrunk, and rates of mutation are much quicker in the virus than in humans, its host. A slow but constant drift of genetic material is on, as is the challenge that faces medical science in the form of new foes.

Some 60 per cent of all infections in humans are because of viruses, the majority of which are undiagnosed. Three-fourths of the total morbidity and half the mortality in India are caused by communicable diseases. WHO has said in its annual report of 1996:

We stand on the brink of a global crisis in infectious diseases. No country is safe from them . . . There are new opportunities for the spread of infection . . . infectious diseases are not only a health issue but also a social one. Until a few years ago, there was optimism—eight out of ten children globally were immunized against half-a-dozen killer diseases. Today, 33 per cent people are dying every year in the world due to an infectious disease.

Much of the character of viruses and bacteria that disease is being defined by what public health experts believe is a social phenomenon. Dr Kalyan Banerjee who headed the National Institute of Virology in Pune for many years has often said that there is a variety of reasons for the way viruses and bacteria change or re-emerge in new forms. A growing population and changing demographic patterns, socio-economic conditions and education, sanitation, food and water supply and general living conditions, are factors that can affect the form that disease-causing organisms take. Changes in the environment—whether global warming or deforestation, overcrowding or changed agricultural patterns—are factors too as are wars, migration and religious beliefs (Banerjee, 1996).

The Burden of Lifestyle

True, social patterns and choices are changing the path of health more than anyone would like to admit. And while the impact is somewhat stealthy and silent in the case of infectious diseases, it is open and tangible when it comes to diseases of the heart, the body's hormone system, cancer, the brain and the nervous system. Lifestyle choices are raising India's burden of non-communicable diseases, and they are catching up quickly with infectious diseases. Hypertension, asthma, cardiac disease, diabetes, paralytic stroke, mental disorder, Alzheimer's disease and obesity, together with TB, malaria, hepatitis and AIDS are fast becoming carriers of death and debilitation for more and more Indians. It is a debilitation that has come gift-wrapped with the techno-savvy, new lifestyles many urban Indians are so proud of today. They are today part of what is considered a globally accepted paradigm of successful modern living, and among them the number of people dying of a heart attack, living with hypertension or diabetes, or having a paralytic stroke has increased. Packed urban lifestyles where stress is king, where being successful means spending as many hours as possible at work, and where choices of unhealthy foods are made all the time, have made diseases that were earlier rare to occur more frequently. The diseases are also afflicting people of a younger age. Ishi Khosla, a consulting nutritionist who runs a health-food shop in New Delhi, has found that though the present generation often continues to eat the kind of food the earlier generation was used to eating, foods like ghee (saturated vegetable oil) for instance, physical activity in the present generation is much less. This has resulted in clogged arteries becoming as commonplace as headaches and fevers. Although major advances in surgical techniques have kept pace with these clogs, clearing them and doing plumbing jobs on people's blood vessels, heart attacks have become a major cause of death in India.

Dr Srinath Reddy, a professor of cardiology at AIIMS, New Delhi, has been examining people's hearts for some years now and what he has found is not good news. Reddy and his team have found that Indians settled in various countries, from the United Kingdom to South Africa, from Singapore to Mauritius, show very high levels of cardiovascular disorders as compared to other ethnic groups. Over the last three decades, rough estimates show that heart disease has grown from a prevalence of 4 per cent to 33 per cent, whereas prevalence of rheumatic heart fever has declined. In the developing world, according to Reddy, 24.5 per cent of all deaths are caused by cardiovascular diseases. That was in 1996 (Reddy, 1998).

Amazingly, while communicable diseases have not really let up in the morbidity they cause, mortality has actually decreased over the years. However, better nutritional standards have led to greater longevity, which in turn has increased the burden of cardiac disease since there are more and more elderly people alive today. It is this transition in demography, accentuated by a shifting lifestyle, that has caused the graph of cardiovascular disease to shoot up. Soon, heart diseases will be the cause of a third of all deaths in India. When Dr Naresh Trehan, one of India's best cardiac surgeons and known the world over for his skills, decided to set up the Escorts Heart Institute and Research Centre in New Delhi, he must have hoped that people would visit the new hospital. But he too might not have anticipated the large number of people, from all over the country, that throng the corridors of this famous hospital.

Going back to Dr Reddy's work, what he has found is intriguing. Some years ago, Reddy and his team observed and studied a group of British Asians and their siblings in Punjab. He found that, in both the groups, Lipoprotein A levels were high, in fact higher than average levels found in Europeans living in the United Kingdom. Lipoprotein A is a lipid-protein that has been associated with an increased risk of coronary heart disease because of its tendency to enhance blood clotting. Lipoprotein A does this by restricting the effective functioning of plasminogen, the body's natural anticoagulant. Other than the similarity in high levels of Lipoprotein A, migrant South Asians had higher plasma cholesterol, body indices and fasting blood glucose levels, lower levels of what is called good cholesterol (HDL cholesterol) and reduced insulin sensitivity, when compared to their siblings living in Punjab. As a result of migration, the adoption of a different lifestyle, and change in food habits, their levels of cholesterol are closer to those of the Europeans whose lifestyles they have adopted. The environmental factors at the root of the weight gain, higher cholesterol, higher blood pressure along with genetic factors like the predisposition to higher Lipoprotein A levels, central obesity and glucose intolerance are causes that are proving to be killers for urban Indians as well who are now succumbing more and more to cardiac diseases.

There are many studies in India that have shown how hypertension, smoking, diabetes and central obesity have emerged as major risk factors in causing a myocardial infarction. Hypertension in fact is a significant disease on its own and is one of the few clear clinical diseases (along with diabetes) that are serious risk factors. In other words, hypertension is a double whammy—not only is the patient suffering from a disease, he/she is also predisposed to a whole lot of other more serious diseases. When R.B. Gaurav and S. Kartikeyan from the Department of Preventive and Social Medicine at the Rajiv Gandhi Medical College in Thane, Maharashtra decided to survey hypertension in an urban slum in Mumbai, their idea was to screen people early enough so that interventions could be planned well in time so as to make a difference. Their study has shown that there are at least 13.9 per cent people aged 35 and above in the slum who are hypertensive (Gaurav and Kartikeyan, 2001). Of the 767 men who were screened, 9.52 per cent were hypertensive, while 18.95 per cent of the 665 women who were screened had high blood pressure. Hypertension, insidious and silently lethal, is really a big health problem across the world. Defining hypertension has always been a sticky issue. But WHO defines it thus: in adults a systolic value of 160 mm Hg or higher, and a diastolic value of 95 mm Hg or higher. On its own, hypertension is often not felt, but it is very vital as a risk factor for cardiovascular complications—cardiac failure, stroke, myocardial infarction and sudden death.

How does one become hypertensive? Experts say it is a combination of environmental and genetic factors. The stress of everyday living and socio-cultural factors are important triggers for hypertension, but a genetic factor is also involved. On an average, hypertension first shows up at the age of 35 and premature death can occur at the age of 50. More than 20 per cent of all cardiovascular disorders in patients who are hospitalized are because of high blood pressure. One of the major disasters that hypertension can cause is paralytic strokes. A stroke can occur in different ways. It could be a thrombotic stroke, or it could be because of a tumour, or an aneurism. In the last two decades, the incidence of stroke seems to have actually declined in the West, simply because of early detection of hypertension, a decline in smoking habits, and control over diabetes (Menon, 1999c). This has not happened in India; in fact more and more young people are succumbing to this terrible problem. With diabetes on the rise, incidents of stroke have also increased because a diabetic patient is more likely to suffer a stroke than a non-diabetic patient. Along with high blood sugar, high cholesterol levels too can make a person vulnerable to stroke. If the blood sugar level is not controlled immediately after a stroke, it can be a really bad prognosis. The key is catching it early: any numbness, even a partial loss of speech, should be attended to immediately. The loss of function that occurs during and as a consequence of a stroke may be transient, or permanent. A stroke often happens very early in the morning, with general weakness, transient numbness, loss of vision in one eye, giddiness, or deafness. Today there are major interventions that can help, specially if the patient is brought in good time. As some doctors say, what happened twenty years ago for the heart is now happening for the brain. Neurosurgeons and other specialists feel that it is high time the 'brain attack' also received the same kind of attention that heart attacks have in the past.

Then there is the mother of all diseases, diabetes. For many diabetologists across India, it is disturbing when they see little children walking into their rooms with distraught parents desperately seeking medical advice. Studies have shown that the age of incidence for this rather impactful disease is slipping all the time (Menon, 1997b). Diabetologists and endocrinologists are worried about the large number of very young (in the 11–16 age group) and obese people who are getting on to their patient lists. This in turn links up with the generally slipping age of disease onset, whether it is hypertension or heart disease, paralytic stroke or diabetes. The problem is that nobody does anything when they see the first signs setting in. A young woman in a clinic in New Delhi was detected positive for diabetes during a pregnancy in 1995, but she did nothing about it. Today, she is being treated for full-blown diabetes. Insulin regulates the body's glucose metabolism and keeps the blood sugar within limits. Diabetes occurs when for some reason the insulin isn't enough or if one's body has lost its sensitivity to the normal levels of insulin. High blood sugar, in turn, can bring with it a long list of problems: that is the over-riding character of this disease. Estimates are that 16–20 per cent of adult Indians who live in cities are diabetic (personal communication with Dr K.S. Reddy, 2001) and very soon the country will have the world's largest number of people suffering from this disease.

Resistance to insulin is linked with central obesity, which is common in India. Close to 30 per cent of urban India is obese. In fact, obesity itself is becoming a big health hazard, as it brings with it a whole list of diseases—diabetes, hypertension, and cholesterol abnormalities that eventually herald heart diseases—which can change people's lives forever.

Of course, obesity can occur for clinical reasons as well. Thyroid gland disorders, for instance, can cause obesity. But one needs no statistics to say that most Indians are obese because they care little about what they eat or how many calories they burn. Between the elevator and the car, the remote control gadget and the computer, physical exercise has taken a backseat. Obesity can be in one's genes, but, as Khosla says, that obesity may be genetic does not mean it is incurable, one can still lose weight if one tries hard enough. Tackling obesity is difficult because it is considered a cosmetic problem, not a health hazard. As long as the machine and the mirror are the focus of weight-loss freaks, the problem will remain. Sadly enough, quick-fix weight-loss programmes have really made a killing over the years. Unless these programmes are backed up with serious lifestyle modifications (exercise and diet) that can maintain a lower weight, most of the lost weight comes back in weeks (Menon, 1996a).

Adding to the Burden

There are many Indians who suffer the agony and incurable pain of Alzheimer's disease. In the many years that V.K. Narayana Menon worked with radio and TV broadcasters, the former Director General of All India Radio had faced a multitude of problems and hurdles. But a sluggish brain was never one of these. Yet, unknown to Narayana Menon, a slow death within his brain had begun when he was in his early seventies (Menon, 1999a). Choked and smothered by protein tangles that refused to go away, Menon's brain cells were dying. He was suffering from the traumatic disease that comes of a shrinking brain—Alzheimer's disease. 'To see him lose his intellect was and is the greatest trauma of my life,' says Menon's wife Rekha. Rekha first figured that something was terribly wrong when one day, their daughter came visiting. He had begun to show memory lapses, but they were written off as natural for his age. This is the problem in diagnosing Alzheimer's disease because its onset is during old age when memory lapses are taken for granted. But that day, after their daughter left in the evening, Menon asked a question that broke Rekha's heart: 'Nice girl, who was she?'

The disease finally took Menon's life. Today there are more than 3 million people suffering from dementia in India but the exact number diagnosed with Alzheimer's disease is unknown. It is in fact considered to be one of the most seriously misclassified and misdiagnosed diseases, and most patients, for no reason, end up in mental asylums. It is a bleak future for these people, as there is no real cure and it is a progressive disease. At the National Institute of Mental Health and Neurosciences (NIMHANS) in Bangalore, figures show that 30 per cent of all dementia cases in India are caused by Alzheimer's disease. The really elderly have a 10 per cent chance of succumbing to the disease, so the numbers are by no means small (Menon, 1999a).

If Alzheimer's is a disease where the care-givers can have an equally traumatic time, then so is cancer. Here is a disease that has also grown—not just because of better detection, but also because of pollution, and new eating habits and lifestyles. Although India does not have as high an incidence of cancer as many other parts of the world, the sheer size of the country's population makes the numbers big and significant. Most commonly, Indian women succumb to cancer of the cervix, breast, oesophagus and oral cavity, whereas men fall prey to oral cancer, cancer of the lung, larynx and pharynx, and leukemia. At least 75,000 new cases of breast cancer alone occur among Indian women each year (Chopra, 2001). It is important to understand that the

National Cancer Registry and hospital-based tumour registries screen a mere 3 per cent of the total population of India. This means that the actual figure of people suffering from cancer is much higher.

Cancer treatment has seen a major revolution in the last few decades, but it is the management of cancer patients and post-remission care that have really changed dramatically. Today, if cancer has lost some of the terrible hopelessness associated with it, it is because of such transformations. Yet, there is little doubt that it is still a disease with almost no cure, and this sets it apart from other diseases and disorders. There are also diseases like asthma, not so totally hopeless as cancer, but associated with a morbidity that can often be very high. In India, 10–12 per cent of the people are asthmatic. Part-genetic and part-environmental, asthma is today managed well as a disease, but can be responsible for the loss of many productive hours for people who suffer the shortness of breath and the wheeze that go with it. Dr S.K. Chhabra has spent many laborious years studying the disease, specially trying to understand its patterns in society, its strong link with pollution, and its prevalence in cities like Delhi. Intending to study the prevalence of asthma in school children in Delhi, Chhabra and his colleagues at the Vallabhai Patel Chest Institute in Delhi surveyed 2867 children between the ages of 4 and 17. Out of the children surveyed, 11.6 per cent said that they were suffering from asthma at that time, while another 4.1 per cent said that they had been afflicted with the disease in the past. This is a high rate, comparable to what is often reported from developed nations (Chhabra et. al., 1998). These scientists underscored what many of us already know about asthma—family history plays a role, yes, but then so does the presence of smokers in the family. Asthma during childhood can take away some of the magic of those young years. Yet, increasing awareness among parents, and better techniques of managing the disease are making it easier for little children who break into a wheeze over pollen, smoke or dust.

When one dwells on the obesity crisis in India, it is difficult to imagine that this is a country where malnutrition is a significant problem, one that has begged for solution over many decades. This is really the most ugly face of human deprivation. Almost 62 million children under the age of 5 are malnourished, and a huge 88 per cent of pregnant women aged 15–49 are anaemic (Haq, 1997). Conditions like anaemia can make life miserable without ending it. Although for the most part malnourishment is a curse the less privileged must carry, the real facts are truly surprising. That is what Shalu Bhargava discovered (Menon, 1999b). Shalu was just as happy as most new mothers, and, of course, tired. That was fine too, everybody told her, delivering a baby and then looking after it was less happiness and more hard work. The backache troubled her as well. Everybody in the family of the thirty-one-year-old Delhi-based woman told her it was normal to end up with an aching back after childbirth, and many pessimistically announced that it would perhaps stay for ever. Then, one cold morning in the December of 1995, as Shalu bent over her baby to change her diaper, she felt an excruciating pain in her back. Around this time, her otherwise normal gait changed to an awkward shuffle, and she knew it was time to take the backache seriously.

Amazingly the X-rays showed nothing. Doctors in some of Delhi's biggest and best hospitals searched tried-and-tested paths—it could be rheumatoid arthritis, or maybe just a bad case of spondylitis (aches and pains of any nature are often categorized as spondylitis)—but were unable to figure out what the real problem was. By now, the young mother was on steroid injections to keep her pain in check. 'You are going to have to live with this condition,' was the cheerful prognosis to a shocked Shalu and her husband, Samir Bhargava, at Chennai's Apollo Hospital, where she was diagnosed as having ankylosing spondylitis. She was heavily dosed with pain killers and was completely immobile by October of 1997, still bereft of a diagnosis. Shalu came face-to-face with a new and traumatic way of life—she could not comb her own hair, she couldn't put on her clothes and she spent long spans of terribly frustrating times in the bathroom, struggling with her pain-ridden, unyielding body. And worst of all, she could not lift her bubbly two-year-old daughter in her arms.

Finally, a day came that would change Shalu's life for ever. She was at the Sanjay Gandhi Post Graduate Institute for Medical Sciences in Lucknow, Uttar Pradesh. Not for herself, for they all thought she was a lost case, but for her husband who was then fighting a rare fungal infection of his adrenal glands. Just as she was wheeled into the foyer, two doctors stared at her and thought to themselves: 'She must be the most chronic case of vitamin D deficiency we have ever seen.' These two doctors, both endocrinologists, were working on an extensive survey of people with bone metabolic disorders and immediately guessed Shalu's problem. Dr Ambrish Mithal, one of the two doctors who had noticed Shalu, diagnosed her as an acute case of osteomalacia, a condition in which the vitamin D in the body begins to corrode the bones. Some months of high-dose injections of vitamin D, and Shalu was picking up her daughter, sitting, standing, walking and laughing like any other woman. Doctors who work on the disease, trying to study its reach, are surprised by its extent in Indian society. In a survey of 800 women from Delhi and Lucknow, Mithal—who now works at the Indraprastha Apollo Hospital in New Delhi—

and his colleagues found a 20 per cent prevalence of severe deficiency of vitamin D, or osteomalacia. It is like a silent, high-morbidity disease, for which till recently there were no proper diagnostic tools available. More than the availability of tools is a lack of awareness among both doctors and patients.

Mithal and his colleagues found that 74 per cent of the women they studied took in just 500 mg of calcium a day, while their requirement is 1000–1500 mg. Little wonder that osteoporotic fractures are four times more common than strokes in India, but the seriousness of it has just not been communicated to the common people in India. Age-related fractures show up much earlier in India (around age 60) as compared to developed nations (around age 80 in the US). As a lifetime death risk, it equals breast cancer. In Shalu's case, the serious deficiency of vitamin D had also affected her ability to absorb calcium. Till the age of 30–35, bone mass grows in the human body. After that, the decline begins at the rate of about 0.2–0.3 per cent a year. This loss increases in post-menopausal women. Fortification with vitamin D is still uncommon in India. Half an hour in the sun is enough for the body to make its own Vitamin D. The human body carries precursors to vitamin D that get catalysed by sunlight to become vitamin D. In India, women often do not get enough sunlight as many of them cover their faces or heads when they get out of their homes. Coloured skin makes the absorption of vitamin D a problem, as a result of which bodies of expatriate Indians living in the US are able to make less vitamin D than those with fairer skins. The real issue is that calcium and vitamin D deficiency are not really recognized as a problem or a disease. Lack of education and the fact that nobody is interested in screening people make things worse. For many nutritionists and doctors in India who deny the seriousness of osteoporosis and osteomalacia, Shalu's is a case in point. She suffered terribly from an illness that had a simple cure, but was just being overlooked—if that is the cost the average Indian has to pay for doctors believing that vitamin D deficiency is not a major problem in India and that it does not cause any serious mortality or morbidity, it is too heavy a cost. Nutritional deficiency in India is a serious challenge to the health system, coming as it does in several forms.

Accepting India's Health Challenges

Disease profiles in India are so complex and diverse that one sometimes wonders how the health system functions at all. Here is a tropical, over-populated country with a lot of infections, lots more diseases and disorders, and little money to face them squarely. Coupled with these are the lifestyle diseases that Indians could well do without but that seem natural fallouts of the urbanization that the country is quickly assimilating as a way of life. Added to this is a lack of information, education and awareness, or even misinformation. The problem is that epidemiological studies and data on various diseases are hard to come by in India; in fact, medical statistics and data records are in a state of total disarray. The three As of medical data—availability, amalgamation and authenticity—are all in such a state that no disease can be truly assessed for its impact and the population that it actually affects. As a result, programmes and policies to tackle these diseases are also faulty and often way off the mark. Surveys and studies are carried out but it takes years for their reports to be finalized, and even when they are final, they are not accessible, more often than not stashed away in some remote corner of a dusty, unenterprising office or library, or buried in the remote pages of some unheard-of journal.

While this cloud of lack of commitment and motivation—on the part of the government, citizens and health experts—gathers around us, the statistics swell, and the list of diseases grows. They seem more than enough for a country grappling with the basics of providing good health care to its people. Even as India struggles to compile and comprehend the masses of ever-growing numbers and data, the disease list is changing its character. Strangely enough for India, what were earlier considered low-key infections of peripheral significance have suddenly taken larger-than-life dimensions, creating new threats to human well-being with higher incidence and prevalence. Meanwhile, the number of people whose health and wellness stand threatened is growing. At one end of the spectrum are complex diseases like cancer and AIDS, with human civilization struggling for a cure, and at the other end are simple, preventable diseases that are wreaking havoc and killing people simply because the government and the society lack the motivation to tackle them and keep them from recurring. Malaria and TB are big villains today, both resurgent and ferocious, and their drug resistant forms are adding a totally new dimension to the treatment of infectious diseases—dimensions that are grave, full of question marks and with few answers from any quarter. This is after early indicators that these diseases were being brought under control. It makes one wonder how the progress of a nation can be defined—is it the growth of its robust software industry or its ability to keep mosquitoes in check or control the spread of age-old bacilli? Infectious diseases, currently, are India's most serious threat. According to WHO, infectious diseases are factors that cause the greatest number of deaths worldwide. Globally, there are some 17 million people who die each year from one infectious disease or the other. At least 7 million of these are from Southeast Asia.

In India, 42 per cent of the deaths that occur each year are because of some communicable disease or the other. Why should these day-to-day, mundane disorders claim lives? Or, for that matter, why should so many of the less-known infections—that is not to say they are less important—raise their ugly heads each year, kill people and disappear, only to resurface year after year? The dengue virus has been able to kill in recent years because the conditions were favourable for the virus to thrive and finally cause an epidemic. This simple circumstance will be found true for most epidemics that occur in India and it shows that citizens will have to take their share of responsibility in controlling infectious diseases. Doctors who try and spread public health messages have said that they find people, who are more-than-ready to gather—with tremendous effort—resources for a vital cardiac surgery, are never ready to pool even a small amount of money for a community health programme, or a neighbourhood sanitation effort that could ensure a reduction in the number of mosquitoes. This attitude has added weight to an already heavy burden of disease, a fact that has made ill health a way of life for countless Indians today.

The BCG Conundrum

The Bacillus Calmette-Guerin (BCG) vaccine is among the first vaccinations that a newborn baby receives. Over the years, India's universal immunization programme has taken the responsibility of vaccinating each newborn child with this vaccine. This is supposed to protect us from TB, at least that is what the officials tell people at the time of vaccinating a child.

What they do not tell us is something that is very important—the real reason why so many Indians still fall prey to TB in adult life. The BCG vaccine, like all vaccines, is given to produce a certain low level of immunity that can protect against a first-time infection with the TB bacillus. The problem is that more than a third of the world is already infected with this bacillus, and BCG cannot protect those who are already infected. That is why experts believe that the contribution of BCG to TB control is very limited, and that the best way out is to rigorously treat those in the community who are already infected (Ten Dam, 1993).

Again, while its larger role may be doubted, the immediate importance of the vaccine in protecting a child from tubercular meningitis and miliary TB is clear. While this is a noble task, it is a fact largely unknown to the average population. Most people believe that the vaccine will shield their child throughout life. It needs to be made very clear that there is no link between the vaccine and adult incidence of the disease. Scientists from the National Tuberculosis Institute under the MHFW in Bangalore carried out a survey on school-going children in the 6–7 age group in Bangalore (Chadha et. al, 2001). They categorized the 94,340 children into two groups—children who had the BCG scar and those who did not. Amazingly, the estimated prevalence of infection was the same in children from both groups. In other words, vaccinated children were at equal risk as non-vaccinated children.

The Woman and the Child:
Fighting for Attention

Serious efforts have not been made to improve the physical, mental, social and economic health of women. In spite of overwhelming constraints, women have struggled to survive, raise children, build homes, provide health care and nurture their families. It has neither been recognized nor appreciated that it is the labour, the perseverance and the caring provided by its women that sustain the world.

—Voluntary Health Association of India (VHAI), 1997

Manju* had delivered her sixth child two years ago—the sixth if you count only the five children who are alive. This slim, good-looking woman is almost accustomed to being pregnant. Just 35 years old, Manju has been pregnant at least eight times in the fifteen years that she has been married, almost once every two years! And it shows—in the way she drags herself up the stairs, in the way her smile has become increasingly tired over the years. Manju and her husband, and now three of their children, work all day ironing clothes in a residential apartment block in east Delhi. It was just a few years ago that things were very different for this young woman who is somehow managing to survive in the shadowy fringes of life in a big city. She had just three children then, the eldest a daughter, and two younger sons. She had much more energy, and life was fun. Now, Manju approaches each day with a fatigue that seems to have grown like a mould over her otherwise radiant face.

'"Why did I have another child?" What sort of a question is that?' is what Manju says light-heartedly when the women, whose crisp cottons she delivers, ask her about her health with genuine concern. Really, why should this 'dhobi' woman, who can barely make her way through the month without borrowing or doing without, have so many children? In Manju's laughter is hidden the real truth—that she has no real answers for why they have so many children. Manju's husband has no answers either. 'Children are the gift of God,' he says, ignoring the fact that it is a hollow sentiment that means little in the harsh reality of their daily existence. It is a tough life; they earn anywhere between Rs 3000 and Rs 5000 each month. Her husband has stuck by her over the years, but he also squanders a lot of money on liquor. Moreover, he beats her when he is drunk and angry. Manju loves her children. So when somebody comments that Manju continues to have children so that she can get them to help her on the job and earn more money, she feels hurt. For she wanted Soni, her eldest, to go to school and do something with her life that was more worthy than just ironing clothes for people. Those were wild dreams even then, and as the number of children grew, the dreams gradually faded into oblivion.

The change in Manju's life has also rubbed off on her children. She has led them into a world where there is never enough food or money or just simple parental love. The school uniforms too have long since come off. Soni has just been married off to an equally young boy from the village, and has come back to be with her mother. It is incredible that two years into Manju's last delivery, she is marrying off her eldest daughter! All at once Soni has started to look very grown-up and now works harder than her mother on the ironing job. Gone is the naughty gleam in her eyes, the impish grin, the jumping and the screeching on the stairs. Soni is now invaluable to Manju who is weakened by repeated childbirth and can no longer carry heavy bundles of clothes. Drained of financial and health resources, Manju and her husband are unable to provide any basic level of nutrition and education to their children. Married so young, Soni will certainly be a seriously anaemic, calcium-deficient woman with many health problems which she will quickly learn to overlook and ignore.

Thoughtless procreation is one of India's most serious health problems, or should one say the fount of many problems. Much of India's population explosion has been caused by people who do not even think before having babies, or do not have the means to prevent pregnancy. These are people who dismiss anxieties about their own health and do not exactly worry about how they will support the extra mouths. Manju is one of the millions of women who do not even question the process of becoming pregnant year after year. What she does not realize, or perhaps realizes but can do little about, is that her constant state of pregnancy is not only a major drain on her own body, but also on the health of her children. Much of this comes from a total lack of awareness and knowledge that a better life does exist, and at no great cost. She is one of the millions of Indian women who have what is technically called an unmet need for contraception, but who will perhaps never assert their inner need to avoid pregnancy. Across India, less than half the population of the country uses any kind of contraception (UNDP, 2002).

Childbirth is amongst the most significant factors that has pushed women—and with them children—towards long-term ill health. This is made all the more complex by social norms, illiteracy and poverty that disallow women from making independent choices. Amongst the most challenging aspects of women's health in India is maternal mortality—the death of women during childbirth.

According to the *Human Development Report (HDR), 2003*, 540 women die per 100,000 live births. This is a depressing scenario because if unwanted pregnancies alone can be taken care of, 25–40 per cent of all maternal deaths can be prevented. Independent studies have shown that almost 18 per cent of total global maternal deaths occur in India. For the 125,000 women who die each year in India during pregnancy and childbirth, the causes are varied, ranging from direct to indirect obstetric reasons. Death could be direct, stemming from haemorrhage, obstructed labour, sepsis, toxemia or unsafe abortions. Of these, post-partum haemorrhage is the most common cause of maternal mortality. There could also be indirect causes such as malnutrition that results in anaemia, or infectious and parasitic diseases like TB and hepatitis. Indian women must be screened for anaemia in a much more rigorous manner than is currently done, and there should be services like immediate access to blood transfusion. Close to a third of all deliveries in India are carried out at home, and even in urban areas a large number of deliveries are carried out in very unhygienic conditions. It is only 42 per cent births that are actually attended by skilled health staff (UNDP, 2002).

Death during childbirth, particularly in this modern age of science and technology, is like the bottom of a dark abyss. But there are millions of Indian women who live suspended somewhere in the middle of this abyss, suffering more morbidity than mortality. Take anaemia, perhaps one of the major factors affecting female health in India, where women record unbelievably low levels of haemoglobin. More than half of India's women are anaemic, and the level of anaemia varies from mild to acute (*National Family Health Survey [NFHS-2], 1998–99*). Studies have clearly shown a correlation between the level of literacy and education and the degree of anaemia, with illiterate women being more prone to anaemia than literate women. A little over half the women in India who get pregnant actually scale down their nutrition status and diet instead of stepping it up (UNICEF, 1996). A woman's body requires five times more iron during pregnancy than normal, especially in the final trimester of pregnancy. That is why anaemia is like a disease in India. The first few years after childbirth are a very serious challenge to women's well-being as they feed and nurture the child through the first and most tricky phase of its development.

But then anaemia is at least a condition that people talk about and discuss. This is more than what can be said for the daily discomfort of reproductive tract infections (RTIs). Millions of Indian women take this discomfort as routine, giving it no thought and, of course, no treatment. It is an established scientific fact that women are more susceptible to these infections than men. RTIs can be classified into three broad types—they may be caused by a sexually transmitted disease (STD); a bacterial infection, either vaginitis or candidiasis; or they may be infections arising from unhygienic delivery practices and a general lack of hygiene. Studies in India have found RTI rates of 52–92 per cent over the years. But the real problem is not the statistic: it is the fact that less than half these women saw it as an abnormal condition that required treatment. RTIs are known to have a very serious long-term impact on the health of the patient, including an increased risk of HIV infection and cervical cancer.

Many women suffer unduly because they end up having children they did not plan to have. If this facet of health care, as also social awareness, could be improved, it would have a dual impact on women's health—one being the most immediate impact of a reduction in the risks of pregnancy and childbirth per se, but the other more important impact would be an improvement in the physical health of women. There is another worrying aspect to the issue of female fertility. A fifth of India's fertility is contributed to by very young women, girls, really, between the ages of 15 and 19. When such young girls become mothers, the infant mortality rate (IMR) is one-and-a-half times more than when women become mothers in their twenties. A total of 37 per cent of the births occur within two years of the previous birth, and this endangers the health of the mother, the infant and its older siblings as well.

This situation in which women find themselves today is in great measure because of illiteracy and a lack of education. In India, only 45.4 per cent women above the age of 15 are literate as compared to the 68.4 per cent of men who are literate in the same group (UNDP, 2002). Till today, even in urban India, girls and boys are treated differently. This strong gender inequity is a major factor that affects the health of both women and children. It emerges in ways dangerous enough to become a matter of life and death for some. A stark index of female health is the sex ratio. Unlike in most other countries, the sex ratio in India has become more and more favourable to males since the early twentieth century (World Bank, 1996). It is 928 females for 1000 males in urban areas, and 957 in rural areas (NFHS-2). Beyond the cold statistic these trends are a reflection of a society in which men are considered the preferred gender, be it with regard to education, health, profession, or general indices of life. A study by the Centre for Enquiry into Health and Allied Themes (CEHAT), an NGO in Mumbai, has shown that morbidity due to health problems is higher in women than in men. The study was done in Nasik, Maharashtra, and recorded an average rate of 569 morbidity episodes per month for 1000 persons. This rate was 330 for men and 812 for women. Some 20 per cent of the morbidity in women was due to reproductive health problems.

For women in traditional Indian homes, one big hurdle is that nobody in the family shows any real concern for their health. Even today, women eat after the men and the children of the family have eaten, and this deprives them of the healthier food items. This may sound simplistic but it is not; it is a vital factor that impacts on the health of Indian women.

Another unfortunate fact is that the family is not always keen to spend money on the health of the woman, and even if some action is taken, the real problem is never addressed. Very often, the real medical problem is skirted and left undiagnosed, and the doctor takes refuge in a diagnosis of 'psychological' or 'psychiatric' disturbance. According to NFHS-2, only a little over half the women in India are involved in taking decisions concerning their own health care. While two-thirds of the women work for money, only 41 per cent of them are free to decide as to what they would do with their earnings. In fact, there is a surprisingly high percentage (18 per cent) of women who shoulder the total economic burden of the family single-handedly.

Why are women dying? Isn't that an important question to ask? The average Indian woman is a hundred times more likely to die from maternity-related causes than a woman in the developed world (World Bank, 1996). Women succumb to illness more than men do, even in a single household (Duggal and Amin, 1989). Community health experts have reason to believe that the discrepancy is less due to biological factors and more due to the fact that the health problems that women face are not given adequate medical attention. This negligence goes a long way in widening the gap. 'In the obsession with meeting family planning targets, training and skill development in clinical diagnosis and rational management of women's health problems have suffered' (VHAI, 1997).

Far away from Manju and her growing family lives another woman. The distance between the two is not geographic, but social. A deep chasm lies between them, but the latter faces a different kind of dilemma. Though she is equipped with the upbringing, education and finances to not make the kind of mistake Manju and her husband have been making over the past few years, she is committing an equally grave mistake. She is trying to choose the sex of the babies she will have. While her education and upbringing allow her to control the number of children she gives birth to, this same background is powerless in the face of societal norms and pressures that make her yearn for a male child. Female foetuses are being hunted out of women's wombs and killed because urban, literate women and the families that surround them are still stuck in a groove. The Pre-natal Diagnostic Techniques Act 1994, has so far failed to deter people from foetal sex determination and selective abortion of the female foetus. Recent pressures from various quarters give hope that something will change, and, for a start, the strictures and penalties have been made clear to people. But any number of rules cannot change societal mindsets, and unless generation after generation of women and men refuse dowry, insist on a good education for the girl child, and learn to demand what is rightfully theirs, change will not come about. Rules on paper often mean little in a country like India. Ten years ago the world got together to create a new agenda so as to make women's reproductive health a totally achievable goal. This was during the Beijing International Conference on Population and Development in 1994. Soon after, the US National Academy of Sciences put together a panel on Reproductive Health in Developing Countries to tackle the 'problem'. Everything was thought out, with emphasis on the prevention of STDs and RTIs. Primary health workers and family planning staff were roped in to help improve the treatment of RTIs at these clinics, sensitize people about the possible complications during childbirth, and spread awareness about and access to contraceptive methods.

Social scientists would like to argue that all this ties up with the cost of having a girl child in an ordinary family. Dowry is an important factor, so is the fact that after all the inputs, the girl child will go away to join another family. Although the urban setting has brought about some change in this perception, widespread transformation is yet to be effected. Even today, parents of liberated, educated young women graduating from the top universities in the country have to arrange for heavy dowries at the time of their daughter's marriage. Across Indian metros, parents of young girls still in high school are happy when they find a 'good match' for their daughters. Often these girls are married off immediately and celebrate their first wedding anniversary with their first child. That this adversely affects women's health is something that both young women and men need to dwell on. Equally, the government must understand that all its policies are pitched against this deeply entrenched system where the girl and the woman will always remain subordinate, and those who break away are labelled rebels.

When Dr Neelam Banerjee and her colleagues at AIIMS decided to interview women seeking abortion, they might have known in some measure what they would find, but the truth sinks in when the real figures stare you in the face (Banerjee et al., 2001). A third of these women went for abortion either because their husbands did not know how to use a condom properly or were unwilling to consider contraception. More than 6 per cent of the women, like Manju, were totally unaware of any methods of contraception. It is this unmet need that fuels abortion as a way out of a sticky situation. Induced abortions were legalized in India in 1971 with the Medical Termination of Pregnancy Act, and since then, the number of legal procedures has reached 600,000 each year (World Bank, 1996). This is again a figure that means very little since illegal abortions abound in India where single motherhood is unaccepted, where a boy child is in greater demand, and where contraception is out of the reach of many for a variety of reasons. There are guesstimates that the actual number of abortions in India could be anywhere between two and ten times this legal number. The real trauma that abortions cause can never be measured in numbers or summed up in a cold graph—it is the trauma caused by a society that encourages young girls and women to end up in abortion clinics run by quacks. It is a trauma that can be weighed by the number of young female lives that are either lost or scarred forever by faulty surgery and treatment.

The high rate of abortions in India is a clear indication that contraception is not as effective as it ought to be. It is ironic that while men take majority of the decisions in most matters in day-to-day life, even in urban Indian society, contraception is an exception. Shying away from the very word, men in India often lay the responsibility for contraception on the woman. According to VHAI, in the 1960s, 11 per cent of sterilizations were tubectomies, but in just three decades this number rose to an enormously significant 96 per cent. To quote from VHAI's report of the *Independent Commission on Health in India* in 1997, 'Every contraceptive, whether old, oral contraceptives, IUCDs, laproscopy, or new, such as depoprovera, NetEn, and even those being researched, such as quinacrine, RU 486, norplant, anti-fertility vaccines, are all targeted at women.' This is also perhaps the reason behind condom use not being as prevalent as it should be. This brings in a whole new set of problems because condoms not only prevent contraception, they also stem the chronic ingress of AIDS by reducing the transmission of HIV. And here is a flip side to the kind of family-planning choices these women make. Across India, more than two-thirds of those opting for family planning have chosen sterilization as the way out, and of these, 71 per cent are women. This means that the use of condoms will be very limited (*NFHS-2*).

Nutrition has also remained a huge challenge for women. Persistent backache has been recorded by women everywhere, especially in urban settings. It is almost like a 'woman's disease' and is often dismissed by the medical profession as non-specific. Backaches are linked to the kind of work the average Indian woman does each day, nutritional deficiency, particularly that of calcium, repeated pregnancies, and a lack of regular physical exercise other than the usual housework. It has often been found that the complaint of recurring back pain is linked to osteoporosis and a chronic deficiency of calcium and vitamin D. However, this is detected only in cases where doctors care to probe beyond the symptom. It is the same case with ill health relating to pre-menstrual syndrome (PMS), a scientifically established condition that requires specific treatment. Thousands of Indian women live through this condition without even knowing that they actually require treatment. Hypertension too has a silent presence among women in India and this is showing up more and more in cities where stress levels have gone up because women have to juggle various roles in society.

That said, there are some signs of hope emerging. This is a transformation that has been catalysed largely by the woman herself, but also by the man. The acceptance by men of the fact that women are equally important in society, and that they need special care simply because of the burden of inequality that they carry as almost evolutionary baggage, has also brought about a change in the condition of women. The modern man is beginning to redefine himself as husband, father and son—many urban men are no longer ashamed of taking on chores in the house, looking after children or nursing their wives during sickness. Even as this transformation slowly begins in Indian society, infants born with low birthweight are still 26 per cent of the total (UNDP, 2002); close to 50 per cent of the children in the 0–5 age group are underweight, and for every 1000 babies born, 69 still die. In the under-5 age group, infant mortality is still 96 out of every 1000 live births. A third of the world's malnourished children live in India. The Indian child is still deeply vulnerable, and carries the tangible impact of the state of women's health.

In Pune, a large and ambitious collaborative study was started some years ago at the KEM, in partnership with the Medical Research Centre (MRC) of the United Kingdom to find out what impact a mother's nutritional status could have on her children. The idea was to explore the child's susceptibility in adulthood to chronic degenerative diseases such as diabetes, hypertension and cardiac-related problems. Dr Ranjan Yajnik of KEM and Dr Caroline Fall of the Environmental Epidemiology unit at MRC conducted the study with funds from the UK Welhome Trust. Studying all the details of the daily diets of 800 pregnant women, the scientists measured and recorded foetal growth, weight gain in the women, and biochemical indicators of nutritional status. Weights of infants and placentas, besides other body measurements, were recorded within twenty-four hours of birth. Women who consumed lots of green leafy vegetables and dairy products as a matter of routine gave birth to bigger babies. A third of the babies were classified as underweight, that is, below 2.5 kg (UNICEF, 1998).

Although the government has made clear its commitment to each child as a matter of policy, providing them nutrition, care and a roof over their heads still remain primary challenges. The Child Survival and Safe Motherhood Programme that was initiated in 1992 has been designed to reduce mortality by addressing the major reasons for morbidity in women and children. There is also the much discussed Integrated Child Development Services Programme (ICDSP), a government programme conducted with World Bank assistance, to improve the status of pregnant women and children below 6 years of age with regard to nutrition and general health. But the reality is that more than 30 per cent of all deaths in India are among children below the age of 5 years (World Bank, 1996). Many never enrol in a school and several drop out at some point or the other—such are the compulsions of ordinary life. While there are stringent laws against child labour, abuse and prostitution, they are one end of the story; the situation on the ground is very different. Even though IMRs have declined over the years, the figures are not very promising. The percentage decline in infant mortality was 14.7 per cent during 1971–81, 27.3 per cent during 1981–91 and 10 per cent during 1991–98. Similarly, mortality declined by 20.6 per cent during 1971–81, by a huge 35.7 per cent during 1981–91, but came down to 15.1 per cent during 1991–98 (*Census of India, 2001*).

The rate of malnutrition is falling, but only at 1 per cent a year, too slow for comfort. Only a third of infants aged 6–9 months are fed complementary semi-solid and solid foods, mostly because few people are aware of the benefits. The decline in infant and child mortality is no longer as rapid as it was in earlier years and a third of all babies born in India today are malnourished. In 1951, infant mortality was 146 per 1000 live births. This came down to 68 in the year 2000. But sadly, the difference is so great between states that averages make little sense. In 2000 the infant mortality was only 14 in Kerala for all 1000 live births, but 96 in Orissa and 85 in Madhya Pradesh (*Annual Report, 2002–03*). According to the government's National Population Policy (NPP), the average IMR in the country should be down to 30 by the year 2010.

It is infants between the ages of 6 months and 2 years who are most vulnerable to malnutrition. This is a time in the child's life when he or she depends completely on somebody else to be fed, a time doctors call the 'period of perpetual hunger'. In fact, a child's health depends almost totally on a mother's well-being, before and after birth. If a woman is anaemic, it affects not just her well-being, but also adversely affects the chances of survival of her unborn baby. A study in a government hospital in Patiala (Iyer, 1998) revealed the impact of the mother's anaemic condition on child mortality. Among women with healthy haemoglobin levels, only 19 infants out of 1000 live births died, while among women with moderate anaemia the figure went up to 49 per 1000 live births, reaching 65 per 1000 live births in women with severe anaemia.

Child health in India is also deeply affected by gender inequality, which in turn affects women's health. So strong are these sex differences that although mortality in infants favours the girl child because the female species has a biological advantage, once the babies grow up the picture changes. According to the *NFHS-2, 50.7* per cent male neonatals die as against 44.6 per cent females; once they cease to be neonatals and till the age of 5, the girls catch up and mortality rates become 26.6 per cent for girls as compared to 24.2 per cent for boys. Given less care, fewer opportunities for growth and development, bound by more rules, girls in many parts of India still have a rough deal.

Women in the reproductive age (15–44) and children below the age of 5 together constitute 36.2 per cent of the population—reason enough that they should be attended to. Although India has a well-chalked-out Maternal and Child Health (MCH) programme, it has often failed to look beyond population control. Ironically though, many of the health problems confronting Indian women could be set right if only they were allowed to bear fewer children. But to be fair, a happy reversal in trends has begun. Back in 1992–93 (*NFHS-1*), each woman on average bore 3.4 children. The *NFHS-2* has shown a decline in this total fertility rate to 2.9 children. This is, of course, still a long way from what would be the ideal (replacement level) of just over two children per woman. What is truly amazing is the difference between regions. Be it women's mortality, literacy or fertility levels, or their ability to make choices, the worst picture emerges from Bihar, Rajasthan, Madhya Pradesh and Uttar Pradesh. Statistics from Kerala, however, read almost like those from an industrialized country. Meanwhile, social norms will be a tougher nut to crack, and while there are signs of change emerging, they are still not significant enough.

HIV/AIDS AND THE INDIAN WOMAN

Almost two decades after the first official HIV infection was reported in India, today, the disease has spread alarmingly in a group of society that was traditionally considered safe: young, married, monogamous women. It is a trend enhanced by the confining social definitions of marriage, lack of choice in protecting themselves from unwanted sexual relations, and the supremacy of the male in a married relationship with many young HIV-positive men not revealing their status to their new wives for fear of being socially stigmatized. There are many women who discover their positivity only once they are well into pregnancy, and often the unborn baby is HIV-positive too. In the major cities of India between 1 and 3 per cent of such women are reported HIV-positive, and in some smaller pockets the infection is as high as 10 per cent in antenatal clinics. But, setting aside the figures, if we step back and view this disease burden against the overarching vulnerability of women in India, it is then that HIV/AIDS becomes all the more difficult for women to handle. Superimposed on existing gender inequality, this most recent disease has created a situation of total helplessness for women. They are stigmatized and discriminated against, and unable to reach out for care and support simply because their spouses are HIV-positive and require all the attention possible, even drugs if affordable.

According to UNICEF, breastfed children of HIV-positive mothers have a 15 per cent chance of contracting the infection. In India roughly two-thirds of young mothers breastfeed their newborns, at least till the child is a month old, if not longer. Programmes are now being introduced by the government to focus on mother-to-child transmission of HIV, and this includes the administration of specific antiretroviral drugs that can reduce the rate of transmission of the virus from mother to newborn during the course of delivery.

But again, some 60 per cent of Indian women have not heard of AIDS (*NFHS-2*). This is an alarming figure that perhaps also explains why there is such a high prevalence of HIV in young and newly married women. Unaware of her husband's sexual history, a woman very often gets infected during the first sexual encounter with her husband. This ignorance finds its worst expression in the transfer of the virus to her baby, which is when she realizes the true import of what confronts her. There are many such young widows in India, struggling to bring up their small, HIV-positive children, anguished by the burden of knowledge that they can neither afford antiretroviral drugs for themselves nor for their little ones; there is also the pain of knowing that they have nowhere to go for support. In most such situations, the blame for the husband's death is also laid at the woman's door, alienating her from family settings and rendering her alone.

Disturbed, Distressed, Damned

Mental illness is not a personal failure. It doesn't happen only to other people.

—Gro Harlem Brundtland, former Director General, WHO, 2001

Have you ever had a chance to sit in the lounge outside a psychiatrist's clinic? If you have, you would know that it is often a crowded place. The small offices of counselors in large city-schools aren't empty either. Then again, ever noticed the alarming statistics of suicides in India? Or of people reporting to doctors with stress, depression, and psychiatric disorders? If you know the answers to these questions, you would also know that depressive disorders are becoming one of the biggest challenges to the health sector in India. In 2001, writing in the *The World Health Report*, former Director General of WHO, Dr Gro Harlem Brundtland said:

Major depression is now the leading cause of disability globally and ranks fourth in the ten leading causes of the global burden of disease. If projections are correct, within the next twenty years, depression will have the dubious distinction of becoming the second cause of the global disease burden. Globally, 70 million people suffer from alcohol dependence. About 50 million have epilepsy, another 24 million have schizophrenia. A million people commit suicide every year. Between 10 and 20 million people attempt it. Rare is the family that will be free from an encounter with mental disorders.

India is no different. Back in 1995, WHO conducted a cross-cultural study in fourteen cities across the world and found that although the prevalence of mental disorders varied considerably, on an average, 24 per cent of all patients studied had a mental disorder. In India, Bangalore was the city selected for the study. It was found that 22.4 per cent of the patients showed mental disorders, the rate of depression was 9.1 per cent, the rate of generalized anxiety 8.5 per cent, and 1.4 per cent showed alcohol dependence. It is with some measure of discomfort that one observes how close the Bangalore sample comes to the world average, where the study samples were from locations as diverse as France, Japan, Brazil, USA, China, Italy, Germany, and the Netherlands.

According to surveys conducted in India, mental disorders occur twice as frequently among the poor than they do among the rich (WHO, 2001). But whether among the poor or the rich, in either case, mental illness is a major burden in India. A study by M.V. Reddy and C.R. Chandrashekhar, who tried to understand the entire spectrum of mental disorders in India, found that neurotic disorders were the most common, occurring in 20.7 people per 1000, followed by all psychotic illnesses at 15.4 per 1000; mental retardation and alcoholism or drug addiction figures were 6.9 each, and epilepsy 4.4 (Reddy and Chandrashekhar, 1998). The amazing thing about mental disorders is their range—from mild, almost undetectable depression to the worst possible condition of mental disability. Anxiety and depression, post-traumatic stress disorder (PTSD), schizophrenia, epilepsy, dementia, substance abuse disorder, and Alzheimer's disease are all different forms of mental illness.

From the diagnosis to the treatment of mental illness, retention of patients in treatment and care is the biggest challenge in India. Stigma and discrimination, a total lack of sensitivity and awareness in society at large, and the actual complexities of treating the mentally sick become major hurdles in the provision of care. Against this social fabric, even the government's programme on paper becomes ineffective. The government had designed a National Mental Health Programme (NMHP) in 1982 which supports twenty-seven district-level programmes in twenty-two states (*Annual Report, 2002–03*). It is apparently meant to ensure that each person has access to basic mental health care, and to work on awareness building in the community with regard to mental health. But the reality is quite different. The National Human Rights Commission (NHRC) has recently found that the state of most mental health institutions is terrible, to say the least (NHRC, 1999). At least a third of the patients suffered from epilepsy or mental retardation and required only specific treatment, not institutionalization. In fact it is well known that such patients do better if they are allowed to stay within their community. Less than a quarter of the many hospitals visited by the NHRC team had trained psychiatric nurses, and less than half had clinical psychologists or specialized social workers. What must this situation be like for those who are financially dependent on state-run services?

Exposed by the powerful devastation only a fire can cause, an asylum in Tamil Nadu's Yerwadi township was an eye-opener to just how bad our health scenario is. In the very early hours of the morning of 6 August 2001, a fire raged through the Moideen Badusha Mental Home in Yerwadi (Kannan, 2002). The people who ran this asylum worked out of thatched huts that resembled cowsheds where patients were housed almost like cattle. This so-called mental asylum was created only because it was located near a religious shrine where devotees flocked to, in search of a cure for 'madness' (Menon, 2001). According to records (Kannan, 2002), people believe that the water at the shrine built around the tomb of Hazrat Qutub Syed Sultan Ibrahim Shaheed Valliyullah (a Moroccan saint who preached Islam during the twelfth century) and the oil that burns in the lamps in the tomb have the power to cure mental illness. However, it has been only a decade since these so-called asylums began to be set up here, usually by people who had themselves been 'cured' of mental illness. In these temporary structures with no basic infrastructure, twenty-five mentally challenged people died that day, chained to posts that prevented them from running.

The only good, if it can be called as much, that emerges from such incidents is that they become a window to the larger scenario. The Tamil Nadu government is said to have quickly taken action, asking for the closure of these homes, and relocating some patients to the Institute of Mental Health in Chennai. Regulations for setting up mental homes were introduced; an unimplemented Mental Health Act (1989) was brought into force with immediate effect, and a Commission of Inquiry was set up to probe the Yerwadi incident. This terrible fire also received national attention, and since then, questions are being raised about the condition of mental care infrastructure in the country. Across India there are thirty-seven mental hospitals owned by the government, and the proportion of mentally challenged people is anywhere between 5 and 10 per cent of the total population of India. There are also 40–50 psychiatric nursing homes/hospitals in the private sector, besides psychiatry departments and wings in medical colleges. According to the government, there are 25,000–30,000 beds available for mentally challenged people (*Annual Report, 2002–03*). We have a health infrastructure that is so inadequate that people requiring psychiatric treatment often do not know where to go. Poverty, combined with blind religious belief, becomes the basic foundation. In addition, these people are drawn into a deep abyss by the staff in these institutions where care and affection for the sick, if it exists at all, is not high on their priority list.

The NHP of 2002 does express the government's anxiety that mental disorders are silent, often not visible or tangible in any society, and more so in India. According to the NHRC, there are at least 20–30 million people who need some sort of mental health care in the country. But somehow, mental illness is still like a silent epidemic. Yet, while mortality from mental illness is not a major problem, morbidity certainly is. The person concerned can lose all quality of life and can also draw with him or her, loved ones, family, and friends. According to the ICMR, though the burden of illness from mental disorders is immense, conventional health statistics tell us very little. The ICMR feels that statistics on mental health disorders have focussed more on mortality, preferring to ignore morbidity and the daily burden that mental disease can become. It is the care and support for the mentally ill that needs to be the focus of all health programmes, not death from mental illness. Mental illness is also set apart from other diseases in that it has complexities that are often difficult to comprehend, even for people who specialize in this area.

Take epilepsy, for instance. It is not one single disease, but a mosaic of many. Few people understand the disorder, and even fewer understand what people go through when in the throes of the awful seizures that characterize the disease.

An ICMR study in urban and rural Bangalore in 1998 found a 0.88 per cent prevalence rate of epilepsy, the worldwide average being about 1 per cent (ICMR, 1998). Effective treatment for epilepsy is so accessible that close to two-thirds of all new cases can be successfully treated as long as the course of medication is adhered to without fail. Drugs to treat the disorder are cheap and freely available. However, the real problem that faces people with epilepsy is the stigma and discrimination that come with it, and this result in many of them ending up in mental asylums where they do not really belong.

Depression—a word that was hardly used some decades ago—is like a living-room expression today, and even ten-year-olds talk about it. In urban India, depressive disorders and anxiety are on the rise, recorded with regularity, and studies have shown how the disorder is being noted increasingly among the poor and among women. It is this rise that is linked to the high rate of suicides in India. According to the 2001 WHO report, over 95,000 Indians committed suicide in 1997, that is one suicide every six minutes. One of every three was aged between 15 and 29. Between 1987 and 1997, the suicide rate rose from 7.5 to 10.03 per 100,000 population. At the time these data were compiled, Chennai had the highest suicide rate of 17.23 among India's top four metros. In fact, suicide is the second most common cause of mortality in young adults (15–35 years). In spite of that, there is no policy or programme for suicide prevention, and there are just 3500 psychiatrists for the country's billion-plus population. The MHFW admits that an inadequate number of specialists is one of the sector's biggest hurdles. Then, of course, the lack of awareness regarding treatment, and the custodial approach to care in mental hospitals are all serious handicaps that are only now being addressed by the ministry. One of the basic pillars of the NMHP is to work on eradicating stigma and protecting people's rights through the mental health authorities of the central and the state governments.

WHO has done a multi-country study on women's health and domestic violence along with the World Studies of Abuse in Family Environments (WorldSAFE) of the International Network of Clinical Epidemiologists (INCLEN) (WHO, 2001). The impact of violent intimate partners on women in various settings across the globe was analysed by asking women whether they had ever attempted or contemplated suicide. In India, 6327 women were interviewed and 64 per cent said that they had contemplated suicide at least once. In fact this figure was the highest, followed by Egypt at 61 per cent, Brazil at 48 per cent, Thailand at 41 per cent, Peru at 40 per cent, Chile at 36 per cent, the Philippines at 28 per cent and Indonesia at 11 per cent. Between 1980 and 1995, suicides had gone up in India by 54 per cent. The overall burden for neuropsychiatric disorders in terms of DALY is projected to increase to 15 per cent by the year 2020, an increase that is proportionately higher than it is for cardiovascular diseases. This increase can be attributed, according to the ICMR, to two reasons: one, that shifting demographic patterns are increasing lifespans and, in turn, the number of people in high-risk age groups. For instance, the number of people with schizophrenia and those with Alzheimer's disease will increase because more and more people in the 15–49 age group are surviving, as are people above the age of 65. The other reason is that there are now so many more reasons for people to be depressed. The ICMR carried out a study of child and adolescent psychiatric disorders in Bangalore and Lucknow. Male children showed 14.3 per cent prevalence in Bangalore and 13.6 in Lucknow, while female children showed 12.6 per cent in Bangalore and 10.6 per cent in Lucknow. The 2001 WHO report has presented selected studies of mental and behavioural disorders in children: in India, in the age group of 1–16 years, 12.8 per cent children were affected, although this was much lower than the 22.5 per cent of affected children in Switzerland (1–15 year olds) (WHO, 2000 and ICMR, 2001).

Another grey area in the realm of mental illness is treatment—is it to be drugs or therapy? What kind of therapy and of what intensity? WHO has noted that some people prefer psychotherapy or counselling to medication for the treatment of depression. Decades of research has shown how specific kinds of psychotherapy (especially those modules designed to be of limited time frame) can be as effective as drugs in the treatment of mild to moderate depression. Studies in India have shown how training general practitioners to provide this care can help make it more effective, and rationalize the cost of treatment as well. 'Open the Doors' is a new global programme to fight the social stigma and discrimination that comes with schizophrenia. In 1999, the World Psychiatric Association launched this programme to increase awareness about the disorder, present treatment options, and to try and improve the attitude of the average public towards the disease. The Indian government has also identified the main barriers to the efficient provision of mental health services: meagre allocation of finances to mental health, shortage of trained psychiatrists, and lack of awareness regarding treatment (*Annual Report, 2002–03*).

At Sneha, a voluntary group affiliated to Befrienders International and based in Chennai with branches in at least ten other Indian cities, there is a helpline for the lonely, the depressed and the suicidal. From 8 a.m. to 10 p.m. each day, Sneha takes calls from at least twenty people. The organization believes that the police records in Chennai city are testimony to what works and what doesn't: since 1989, suicide rates have dropped dramatically in the city. Befrienders International is working in more than forty countries across the world to help people on the verge of suicide. Whether through a phone call, a letter, or even face-to-face interaction, volunteers are trying to break the awful circuit of thought and action that leads people to suicide. And if it works, nothing like it. As the 2001 WHO report says:

> The time lag between initiation of actions and their resultant benefits can be long. But this is an added reason to encourage all countries to take immediate steps towards improving the mental health of their populations. For the poorest countries, these first steps may be small, but they are nonetheless worth taking. For rich and poor alike, mental well-being is as important as physical health. For all who suffer from mental disorders, there is hope; it is the responsibility of all governments to turn that hope into reality.

IS THERE A WAY OUT?

According to WHO (*The World Health Report*, 2001), there is a path that one can follow to make things better not just for the mentally sick, but also for human society at large. Recommendations, we know, can remain just that and nothing else. Yet, in the simplicity of these recommendations of the WHO is reflected the truth that change is just round the corner. The will to change, though, is always a little farther than that.

1. Provide treatment in primary care: Train general health personnel so that more and more people can get easier and faster access to services. The current scenario is such that mental health care is so specialized and so much in a niche of its own that not only is it inaccessible to many, it is also under a heavy social label, besides being ridden by non-specific and inappropriate treatments.

2. Make psychotropic drugs available: These medicines should be included in the essential drugs list of each country and should be made available easily. Although such drugs are the accepted method of first-line treatment, their non-availability is a big hurdle.

3. Give care within the community: A mentally ill person will almost certainly be better off being cared for by his or her own community, rather than being institutionalized. It is time to strengthen and enable the community so that it can provide the best possible care to its mentally sick. If the large, impersonal hospital could be replaced by community-based, intimate service, care for the mentally sick might be both cost-effective as also of a quality that would show respect for basic human rights, something that is constantly violated in the current scenario.

4.   Educate the public: This is vital to bust the deep-rooted myths that surround mental disorders. If society at large could become more aware of the kinds of mental disorders, treatment options, recovery paths and the basic rights of people with such disorders, mental health services would become much more effective. This, WHO believes, would to some extent bridge the chasm between mental and physical health care.

5.   Involve communities, families and consumers: If this happens, services would be better tailored to meet the needs of people, and would become more effective in meeting their goal.

6.   Establish national policies, programmes and legislation: Genuine and effective action to improve mental health services will be impossible without a strong mental health policy, and government-based programmes and legislation. More importantly, they should be designed according to the current scenario, keeping modern needs and human rights in mind. Budgets across the world are low as far as mental health care goes.

7.   Develop human resources: The training of mental health professionals is at present very inadequate in many developing countries across the world. Health professionals should not only be trained adequately, they should also be encouraged to stay on in their country and work. Teams of specialists in mental health care, including psychiatrists, clinical psychologists, psychiatrist nurses, social workers and occupational therapists should be built up at the secondary health-care level.

8.   Link with other sectors: Sectors like education, labour, welfare, and law should be involved in providing mental health care to the community. This will make the whole process more effective.

9. Monitor community mental health: Health information systems should include mental health in their scope. Determining trends in mental health, detecting problems and working on more general measures will not just allow assessment of health programmes and their effectiveness, but will also help in planning more targeted interventions.

10. Support more research: Mental disorders have been a constant challenge to the medical scientist, and will continue to remain so. Building the capacity of developing countries to conduct mental health research will be vital in preparing better and more effective interventions.

In Deep Slumber, Or Just Waking Up

Urban health care is in a total state of anarchy today with almost no regulation of the private sector.

—K.S. Reddy, Professor of Cardiology, AIIMS (personal interview)

Service providers of health care in India are facing the biggest challenge ever in the history of their existence. Across the country, cutting across societal and economic borders, the burden of disease is higher than ever before. Within the existing infrastructural and policy-based dimensions of the governmental system there are enormous strengths in the form of specific programmes, policies, institutional guidelines, full government departments with clear mandates before them, and an enormous network of hospitals, health centres, doctors and paramedical staff—all created to make the delivery of health care efficient, and people-friendly. The problem is that it is a system on standby. Although this extensive public health infrastructure has been building up over the years since Independence, the quality of these basic services has deteriorated extensively and has begun to leave an impact on the lives of people. A change in the situation seems almost impossible unless there is a health revolution, as there has been with saving the environment or with agriculture.

Cashing in on this near-total collapse of the government-owned health-care network, the private sector has experienced a phenomenal boom and health care is now big business. Hospitals have come to resemble five star hotels, as do the medical bills! In stark contrast to the amount of money being poured in to the private health-care sector by entrepreneurs, the government's spending on health is abysmal—the public health necessities of each Indian cost the government an amount that would put anybody to shame—Rs 200 a year! Ironically, the seriousness of the rot in the system has been admitted by the health authorities themselves. The *NHP, 2002* makes no bones about the current state of affairs of the health infrastructure of the country:

> Despite the impressive public health gains, there is no gainsaying the fact that the morbidity and mortality levels in the country are still unacceptably high. These unsatisfactory health indices are, in turn, an indication of the limited success of the public health system in meeting the preventive and curative requirements of the general population.

With a badly under-financed public health system on the one hand, and a private health-care infrastructure that is still in great measure unaccountable but is being increasingly used by all, it is difficult to imagine the country being able to rise to its ever-growing health challenges (Peters et al., 2002). The NHP of 2002 has not minced words about the situation in which India's health-care infrastructure is today. Both out-patient and in-patient services are suffering because of inadequate funding, obsolete equipment, dilapidated hospital buildings, a scarcity of essential drugs and consumables, a scanty population of doctors and paramedical personnel, over-crowding and a very low quality of service.

While it is undisputed that the more proactive approach would be to address the rot and try to find solutions to rise above it to rebuild and revitalize the system, it is also important to understand the factors that have led a health system, which was once characterized by strong infrastructure and sufficient policy initiatives, to the disorder it is in today. Put simply, public health care in India is cash-strapped, the existing infrastructure and programmes are grossly mismanaged, and policy initiatives, with a few exceptions, have remained paper tigers. There is also a strong pull-down factor that emerges from the erosion of ethics and motivational medical practice among doctors and in health institutions today, but this latter aspect has much more to do with human nature than with infrastructure. This erosion and the significant contribution it has made towards the disintegration of the public health-care system will be discussed in Chapter 5. While it would be futile to contemplate whether the root cause of the rot is the crumbling infrastructure or the collapse of ethical medical practice, there is no doubt that the system is in peril. So, if the management of existing infrastructure and programmes, strong health budgets and the effective implementation of policy initiatives are to be placed at the hub of what is currently playing out in the health sector in India, would one want to attach a priority listing to each of these factors? Perhaps not, because each one affects the other. Infrastructure cannot be managed efficiently without sufficient money or strong policy. At the same time, lack of funds should not become an excuse for malfunctioning infrastructure and programmes. But yes, it can be said that mismanagement of what already exists as a network of institutions, individuals and strong health programmes is really the most significant drawback of the health-care system because it nullifies any reform that may emerge, either in the form of fresh budget allocations or changes brought about in the government policy.

Mismanagement, India's Bugbear

WHO understands the organization of health systems as three fundamental forms—the bureaucracy, a long-term contractual arrangement, and short-term, market-based interactions. According to the WHO, India is one example of a nation that has all three forms: the government, the private practitioner, and the partnership between the public sector and non-governmental organizations (NGOs). Is this a strength that India is not using adequately, or is this what creates the chaos and the directionless movement? Many critics would point to the latter. The network of primary health-care centres (PHCs), which was in the early decades of Independent India a showpiece of sorts, has all but collapsed. Relics and remnants of these centres can be seen as one travels around the country—ramshackle dispensaries where no sensible human being would want to enter, let alone put his or her life in the hands of those who run such centres. Estimates of the government of India show that the country has a shortfall of about 16 per cent in the number of PHCs and community health centres (CHCs). The same shortage is as high as 58 per cent when only CHCs are considered. Shortage of staff and drugs makes the going even harder. While this network has serious inadequacies in terms of actual resources and physical infrastructure, an equally acute problem is getting good, qualified medical doctors to serve in these clinics. This is a serious problem that is affecting the efficient management of the network. For most young doctors who graduate from medical colleges, serving in these centres is almost like a punishment to be avoided in any possible way. This is a problem the government is clearly aware of, as is evident in the NHP, 2002: 'No incentive system attempted so far has induced private medical personnel to go to such areas; and even in the public health sector, the effort to deploy medical personnel in such under-served areas has usually been a losing battle.' This scene plays out not just in the rural outback, but also in those ignored sections of big metropolises that almost seem to fall off the fringes. Revitalizing the management of the primary health-care network may be a cost-heavy option, but one that cannot be ignored.

The malaise that has overtaken medical infrastructure is everywhere and for all to see, but if there is one place that serves as a glaring example of this malaise it is an institution called the Medical Council of India (MCI). It is located in a quiet by-lane of central Delhi, close to the corridors of power. For many years it remained a shabby, derelict building that begged to be ignored completely if one passed that way. Chances are, many people in Delhi have never seen it. The MCI was established almost seventy years ago with the far-reaching and significant function of 'establishing uniform standards of higher qualifications in medicine and recognition of medical qualifications in India and abroad' <http://www.mciindia.org>. Involved closely with the registration of medical professionals, and the overall responsibility of giving clearances for the setting up of medical colleges and institutions across the country, the loftiness of the MCI, unfortunately, ends there. The dereliction that showed in the building is just the outward, physical reflection of a much more serious concern: the culpable negligence that is, in no mean measure, responsible for the condition of health care in India today.

The MCI is responsible for the 'maintenance of uniform standards of medical education, both undergraduate and postgraduate; recommendation for recognition/de-recognition of medical qualifications of medical institutions of India or foreign countries; and the permanent registration/provisional registration of doctors with recognized medical qualifications'. Unfortunately, the MCI too is a mismanaged dinosaur and although its mandate includes overseeing the medical profession in India, its officials rarely act unless a complaint is actually lodged with them—proactive policing, obviously, is not their cup of tea. The MCI does not work on the premise that the law of the jungle currently prevails in the medical profession and it still functions on the age-old 'nobility' factor. It is an organization which had always maintained that it only registered doctors for medical practice and had no other role to play. For countless people involved with the MCI in one way or another—doctors, lawyers, educationists and activists—this laxity in approach has been a major source of anxiety. But now, the mismanagement stands challenged. The year 2001 changed the course of the relentless malingering that had become a way of life at the MCI. Dr Ketan Desai, the MCI's erstwhile president and a powerful and rich doctor from Gujarat, came into the public eye as a result of a case in the High Court of Delhi. Challenging Desai's office as president, a writ petitioner had forced public attention on the continuing bribery, misuse of official powers and repeated indulgence in varied corrupt practices by Desai, and also by the MCI under his stewardship.

It was this legal backing that vindicated the unproven doubts many people had about the working of the MCI. The institution's real mandate, its genuine duties, and the corruption within have always been a cause of anguish. Now, with changes at the helm there is hope that the MCI will become a better place. But many years of indifferent administration of an institution that could otherwise have been a source of inspiration for the profession have made the MCI one of the best examples of what exactly is happening in the Indian health-care sector—a deep slumber, or worse, mismanagement and misuse of power, and a total lack of motivation among officials who are the chosen administrators of this crucial sector that controls and influences the health of every average Indian. These become acts of offence when their impact on people's health is actually felt. It is time the health infrastructure came under stringent regulation and was forced to perform to the best of its ability.

It is this infrastructure—lying as it is in different stages of degradation or slumber-filled inactivity—that serves as a backdrop against which India's multitudinous health-care programmes play out. According to the VHAI, while many new programmes have been launched in the country over the past several years, they are narrow, concentrate on individual diseases, and have not been integrated into the mainstream, existing infrastructure. These factors cast a shadow over their lasting success. India's failure to control communicable diseases like TB and malaria mirrors the state of the system, and it is a failure for which many innocent people are paying dearly, often with their lives. And, even as the government struggles with these diseases, their drug-resistant forms have taken root (see Chapter 1), placing greater challenges before an already sagging system. To anybody who would care to take a critical view of the huge burden of disease due to TB or malaria, mismanagement would be uncomfortably evident as the major reason why these diseases still remain so prominent in India's burden of ill health. The RNTCP has seen some success but there is still a long way to go. That TB has made a comeback is a frustrating reflection of how public health programmes have been disintegrating in the country. It took the country too long to create a programme whereby the drug intake for curing TB could be monitored and ensured. As for malaria, the irrational use of DDT and the lack of basic sanitation and hygiene, besides lack of awareness among the people, have led to a huge increase in the incidence of this disease through a resurgence of the mosquito population across the country.

India has a heavy burden of leprosy: 60 per cent of all leprosy patients across the world live here. In fact, the entire global spread of active leprosy is clustered in just a dozen countries of the world. There are anywhere between 350,000 and 500,000 leprosy patients in India, and in one year (2001–02) close to 62,000 new cases were detected. It was hoped that by 2000 the incidence of this dreaded disease would fall below 1 per 10,000 people, as recommended by WHO, but the current rate is 4.2 cases per 10,000 (*Annual Report, 2002–03*). A global programme spearheaded by WHO took off in 1991 and elimination levels were reached in more than 100 countries. The second phase of a World Bank project, aimed at eliminating the disease by 2004, is still underway, but the disease still shows endemicity in eight states: Uttar Pradesh, Bihar, Orissa, Madhya Pradesh, West Bengal, Uttaranchal, Chattisgarh and Jharkhand. This challenge may be bigger than it seems. The government's judgement is that the programme is on track and if the burden still exists, it is because the disease has been around 'for centuries in this vast country' (*Annual Report, 2002–03*).

Ironically, the government sometimes takes decisions that reverse the extraordinary success of good intervention programmes that are up and running, almost to the extent that it appears as though success does not hold much meaning in the health sector. Here is an example of a programme where disaster almost struck, but timely intervention from learned bodies was able to set it back on track. In 1984 it was found that the only way to effectively tackle iodine deficiency disorders (IDDs) was to iodize all salt for consumption. As recently as 1998, the government formalized a ban on the sale of non-iodized salt. Iodine deficiency can result in unsafe pregnancies and the birth of deformed babies with low levels of intelligence. Armed with this knowledge—or so one thought—the government imposed this ban; in May 2000, however, it decided to withdraw the ban (Menon, 2000). It was reported that a group of Gandhians from Gujarat had pleaded with the former prime minister Atal Bihari Vajpayee to allow every consumer to make a free choice of whether or not he or she would like to consume iodized salt. The government went to the extent of seeking an amendment in the act that banned the sale of non-iodized salt, despite the fact that in its own records it admits that IDDs in the country has declined significantly since the universal salt iodization programme was started. The real reason behind the proposed amendment was that since the ban was enforced, 6000 small salt manufacturers had gone out of business as they had not put in place the iodization process in their manufacturing plants.

The late Professor V. Ramalingaswami, former Director General of the ICMR and one of India's best-known medical experts, had said that it was regrettable that the government debated lifting the ban, since India was very close to its goal of eliminating IDDs. He said that it was perhaps only another year or two before the entire population would begin to get iodized salt. Serious IDDs dog the Kangra valley in Himachal Pradesh. The water there has no iodine and the consumption of iodized salt is the simplest possible health intervention. As Professor Ramalingaswami said, 'There is no public health measure as safe and simple as the addition of iodine to salt for human consumption.'

If this is the case, why would a successful programme be tampered with? Or, more importantly, why not prioritize action and address non-performing programmes instead of unnecessarily upsetting successful programmes? There will be no answers to this, of course. And anyway, going by the current levels of awareness, it is difficult to see the average Indian making conscious, informed choices regarding the kind of salt they will consume, when something as basic as condom use still remains an issue.

Talking of condom use, this small and simple intervention that can make a difference between contracting HIV and remaining safe from the killer disease has been in the eye of a storm. With frequent changes at the helm in the MHFW, a shift had taken place in the HIV/AIDS prevention programme to make it less condom-centric. Abstinence, safe blood practices and other measures have been highlighted. Just when people across the country were beginning to accept condom use as something that did not diminish the sexual experience, and as a practice not to be shied away from, this shift in the programme in 2003–04 was significant. AIDS is a disease around which India needs to build a strong prevention programme since it is certainly not a disease we can afford to cure as of now, nor is there a foolproof cure. For an average Indian, the package of antiretroviral drugs can only spell financial ruin, with a month's dosage costing a minimum of Rs 2000 for one person—almost a single Indian's monthly salary in many families. Although there are around 5 million Indians infected with HIV, awareness levels are poor and the infrastructure still does not offer a specific testing or treatment regime to all. As a result, most people do not even know that they are HIV-positive (Pallikadavath and Stones, 2001). There is a large section of the population that is still unaware of the disease, the methods of prevention, and ways out for a person who becomes infected with HIV. While awareness generation is a big component of the programme, it is still far from being adequately spread in the right manner and for the right target audience. At this juncture, a confusing message from the top echelons can be disastrous and may have far-reaching, negative consequences. Despite the well-known fact that 85 per cent of the transmission of HIV in India is through the heterosexual route, the rationale of saying that condoms are not the most important safety measure is incomprehensible. This short-sighted governmental approach has left its mark.

Many public health programmes lack detail in their planning. Little wonder that efficient and forward-looking management in the health sector is a matter of big concern. This cuts across different fields, whether vital or marginal. In fact, daily managerial issues are also causing a lot of slowdown in the way health programmes are run. A lack of communication and interaction between various arms of the government is affecting the proper outreach of quality health services. That medical professionals from highly specialized fields are heading public health organizations is another factor. Here is the blatant truth: many people see public health as a very broad discipline in which anybody can become a specialist, in the belief that it is simply about clean water and throwing garbage in the right place. Nothing could be farther from the truth. If anything, there is a real and overwhelming need to groom and foster a crop of specialized public health experts. This is not to say that there are currently no experts, but much stronger roles are needed to be defined for them. The way public health is taught needs refurbishing as well. A network of existing institutions will become necessary and a common curriculum might make sense, supplemented with inputs from various institutions on special subjects.

Then, of course, the issue of mismanagement perhaps comes through the strongest if one considers the billion-plus population of India, and very little resources to support them all. Back in the 1970s, the population control programme was actually working. But then the government decided to switch to a non-target approach. The population, meanwhile, has grown and although fertility rates are on a slow decline, it is still too early to say whether this is good news or not. The country's unmet need for contraceptive choices is a clear example of bad management of a situation, and there is still a long way to go before this reality changes for the better. And if abstinence among the average population were to work—as suggested by the government in response to checking HIV/AIDS—India wouldn't have had a population problem.

The polio control programme is also fast attaining the dubious distinction of not working—something, somewhere, is going terribly wrong. The WHO has expressed concern about a resurgence in the incidence of polio in the country (Ravi Kanth, 2003), highlighting the fact that a significant cutback in the number of immunizations has caused a 'phenomenal rise in polio cases and the re-establishment of transmission in previously polio-free parts of the country'. Polio has resurfaced in ten states, and almost 65 per cent of the global burden of polio is in Uttar Pradesh. Health experts guess that the efficiency of immunization has suffered because of a fatigue among workers, and because of the ineffectiveness of the vaccine in some cases.

Unscrupulous practices—growing unchecked—are also affecting health outcomes. When dropsy affected many people across northern India in 1998, the Prevention of Food Adulteration (PFA) section of the government was caught napping. Mustard oil, made out of mustard seed stock that was highly adulterated with seeds of a plant called argemone, was being sold everywhere, put out in the market by unauthorized manufacturers who were fearless of the law. After the first few cases were diagnosed, a public fear rang out. All of a sudden, labs sprouted everywhere and people were talking about test tubes and lab tests and poison in their oil. The PFA had more excuses than answers for what was going so terribly wrong, while people suffered painful symptoms of the adulteration. Its officials say they are constantly busy doing random tests of food items, picking up thousands of samples, from masalas to processed foods and everything else we eat. It has been established beyond doubt that the fifty-odd deaths at that time, and the hundreds of people who had to suffer various degrees of pain from the adulteration, were caused by deep-rooted corruption, malfunctioning or non-functional labs to check adulteration in foodstuff, and an overarching and massive regulatory failure (Menon, 1998).

Mismanagement of the sector is also evident in the way blindness is being tackled. The government has been running a National Programme for the Control of Blindness for more than twenty-five years but the burden of blindness is still significant. Take the case of eye camps held year after year in cities, towns and villages. It is almost like the classic village fair. The removal of cataract is a fairly minor and regular surgical procedure, but sheer mismanagement can put eyesight at a premium for these people (Chapter 5). Most of the people blinded are poor, with little power or privilege to carry their complaint further and seek justice. And what about eye donations? In neighbouring Sri Lanka it is mandatory to donate the eyes of the dead; in fact the entire world depends on this small island-nation for eyes. It is almost an industry and a single eye can cost up to Rs 5000.

Ms Tanuja Joshi, who has worked for years towards making eye donation an easy exercise in India, throws up her hands in despair. Here's the reason for her despair: some 8 million people die each year, but the number of eye donations is only a few thousands. Working for the Venu Eye Centre in New Delhi, Joshi has found that most of the people who actually donate their eyes are from the working middle class. Joshi also works closely with the Eye Bank Association of India (EBAI). Basing all their work on the fact that eyes can never be bought for money and can only be a gift, the EBAI has been relentlessly pursuing the task of getting people to pledge their eyes for removal after death. Yet, with the general lack of awareness among people, the number of pledged eyes is inordinately more than the actual number of donations when the need really arises. With religion coming in the way, relatives of the deceased, who had pledged his or her eyes, will often not inform or allow eye-bank officials to take away the donated eyes in time. And it is a short window of opportunity—a couple of hours, when the eye as an organ still remains viable and capable of further use. The government does not really monitor eye banks and there is a scarcity of good hospital-based eye retrieval programmes whereby young and sudden deaths can also become sources of eyes. And the clincher is that more than two-thirds of blindness in India can be cured with good corneal transplants. There are numerous unclaimed dead bodies across the country, but they do not translate into hope for the blind, which was the original spirit of eye donation. This is because of all the hurdles that exist between the pledging of eyes by a potential donor and the actual donation process. So, donations are all very well, as are all those signed forms and advertisements, but the huge managerial hurdles, between that emotional statement and those eyes really being put to use, are considerable and yet unresolved.

Looking beyond the problems of managing the physical infrastructure, a primary challenge that emerges is the lack of rigour in the health system's approach to statistical data on diseases, medical practices and health problems. More than half a century of Independence and India still does not have a good statistical database of diseases and disorders that affect Indians each day. The country's fairly large institutional base (research institutions and hospitals) has failed miserably in its inability to create a reliable pool of authentic, up-to-date and exhaustive data on illnesses in the country. Whatever little is available is not just hard to get but also often so late in being released that the numbers become hopelessly outdated. Ambitiously, the NHP of 2002 hopes to put in place a modern and scientific database of health statistics of India. Although not enough can be said about the value of such a database, the reality is that after so many years of negligence it is not going to be easy. But if it happens, it would indeed be the best thing for the health-care sector of the country.

Mismanagement has also plagued the human resource sector that fuels the health-care system. There is cause for concern in the knowledge that while 15,000 doctors get a medical degree each year, there are some parts of the country where there are no doctors at all. There is need to worry about medical research priorities, especially because past exercises in trying to analyse these priorities have drawn a dismal picture of what medical science is really researching in India and what the person on the streets needs from this researcher in real terms. Are sufficient research efforts being made to solve small, but important, problems like ARIs and diarrohea? Is there any strong body of research that is working out public health goals and methodologies for the years ahead? Students studying to become doctors in premier medical colleges and universities rarely care or know much about public health. Community and public health are not fashionable streams in medical colleges. Some of the biggest public health institutions are not in good health themselves, and this is a major factor in the lack of success of public health programmes in the country.

The Roar of the Paper Tiger

At the core of any reform to revamp the health-care system is health policy. The governmental system, crammed as it is with policies and declarations, still faces one supreme challenge—of having all those good-sounding words jump out of files and books to become functional in the real world. It is almost too much to ask for. For the many who have heard of Alma Ata, the separation between the words in declarations and the real situation will be clear. In 1978, several countries of the world met in this city in the erstwhile Soviet Union as part of a global initiative to push for health action and research across the world. As part of the Alma Ata Declaration, 'Health for all by the year 2000' was to be ensured by all signatory countries, and primary health care was to be the priority. India was a part of this declaration. Since then, many declarations have been announced, many signatures have been scrawled across lofty policy decisions and goal settings. Today, 'Health for All' is not even mentioned in the approach paper to the Tenth Five Year Plan (Seetha Prabhu and Selvaraju, 2001), and most of those for whom the phrase was meant are still waiting. But many are also watching. The system, with its great propensity for paperwork, exciting policy documents, and meaningful debate and discussion, needs to rise above the government files and show it can work. Take the NHP itself, which sets out an ambitious charter. But, on the ground, hardly anything is followed up and the papers become almost immaterial. This is perhaps India's biggest and most problematic malaise: solutions are worked out, but remain back-of-the-book calculations with little done in reality. Action does take place, but a little too late, and the delay makes the solution obsolete.

It was in 1983 that the NHP was last formulated before its current version. The ministry makes no bones about the fact that while some of these policy initiatives taken almost two decades ago have shown results, several have been complete failures. The Eighth Five Year Plan reiterated this, and the Ninth Five Year Plan had this line hidden away somewhere in the document: 'the essential inter-linkages between health services delivery and health manpower development are still not fully understood and operationalized.' Over the decades, many committees have made recommendations, but implementation has always been a serious issue that has adversely affected health-care systems and their efficiency (For further information see Box: List of Recommendations, pp. 95–96).

Many policy decisions and pronouncements have never seen the light of day after they are painstakingly formulated and written and made much of in press conferences, workshops and government committees. The acceptance of the Calcutta Declaration on Public Health in the year 2000— a joint effort by WHO and the government—was supposed to provide a great impetus to the way public health was being handled in the country. Its expected outcome was to create awareness, 'develop strategies to promote partnerships and further strengthen public health policy and practice in the countries of the Southeast Asian region'. But that was four years ago, and results are yet to become visible. It had high-sounding goals of promoting, among other things, supportive environments, community participation in health programmes, careers for public health professionals, and a recognition of the need to establish a separate cadre of public health professionals while calling for a total restructuring of the public health system. Four years down the line, the suggested changes have remained good ideas on paper. The Declaration itself says: 'We urge all member countries as well as the WHO to . . . jointly advocate and actively follow up on all aspects of this Calcutta Declaration on public health.' But, lack of action in India as a follow-up to paper policy has disillusioned ordinary people. There is a sense of loss, because back in 1946, when the Bhore Committee Report was released, it established that the initiation of a health-care system would be with the formation of a solid primary health-care sector and that every Indian should be able to access this primary care regardless of economic strength (For further information see Box: List of Recommendations, pp. 95–96). In fact, this report was an important reason for India's all-out support to the Alma Ata Declaration (Peters et al., 2002). That was then, and this is now.

Where is the Money?

Indian democracy has seen many political parties come and go. For all of them, investment in health has been a secondary consideration. In fact, India spends less than almost all other countries, even less than the poorest African nations, on health care. It is almost a joke, really, that India is placed among the lowest 20 per cent spenders among nations (Peters et al., 2002).

The budget of 2002–03 too fails to fill—in any tangible manner—most of the gaps that already exist. Investment in public health has declined from 1.3 per cent of the GDP in 1990 to 0.9 per cent in 1999. According to the *NHP, 2002*, 'The central budgetary allocation for health over this period, as a percentage of the total Central Budget, has been stagnant at 1.3 per cent, while that in the states has declined from 7 per cent to 5.5 per cent.' Well, who decides these swings in public spending? The government, of course, which is why many experts believe that nothing is going to change without macroeconomic reform. There is also a lot of variation between states: Kerala, Punjab and Tamil Nadu, for instance, spend double the amount that the governments of Bihar and Madhya Pradesh do on each person's public health-care needs (Peters et al., 2002). So there rests cold, sterile statistics— figures you wish you could ignore. But that is not possible for they are the result of decisions taken by the government. What of the millions of Indian women who still die while in the throes of childbirth? Why is diarrhoea still a major cause of death among children? Why should so many Indian children go blind? These are facts that hold a mirror to the total apathy and lack of dedication to the health sector, one that should actually command maximum attention. There are lots of people out there dying of health problems that should not be a threat today. Excuses for this obvious laxity abound, and the biggest one is that India spends so little on health care.

As has already been mentioned, the amount spent on each Indian by the government as public health expenditure is so low that it is almost close to nothing. Overall investment in health care by the state has been declining, as can be seen in a decline in capital expenditure (Duggal, 2001). In fact the *NHP, 2002* says: 'The current annual per capita public health expenditure in the country is no more than Rs 200. Given these statistics, it is no surprise that the reach and quality of public health services has been below the desirable standard.' This dwindling financial commitment to health-care spending raises questions about the progress of a nation. There is global acceptance of the fact that the world's changing economic scenario is creating a negative impact on health. This acceptance has led to partnerships between nations and between governments and multilateral agencies in an effort to bolster support for health programmes. India has been no exception, with the government managing to put together enough funds from international donor agencies (WHO, 2000). Out of the allocation of Rs 30 billion for health in the Ninth Five Year Plan, Rs 18 billion was from external funding.

But, such funding has a flip side as well. Many public health experts feel that heavy donor funding in small areas for specific projects can often have the island effect—that is, a small, restricted area flush with funds, and a project that cannot be replicated simply because such a high level of funding can never be sustained. The WHO says that donor contributions are of great importance and that donor funding can play a key role in the financial allocations for health programmes in developing countries (WHO, 2002). India has been the recipient of large, absolute amounts of such funding in recent years. The WHO report is however critical of the procedure such funding mechanisms follow, which is through independent projects between donor agencies and the specific national institution. With negotiations for such projects being constricted, there is often a duplication in programme design, and there is a need to create nodal agencies for wider, long-term support to programmes of a larger scale. Then there is a whole array of large, international organizations doing what is considered advisory work. Whether it is WHO, or UNICEF or the United Nations

Development Fund for Women (UNIFEM), these organizations have a significant presence in India, and while they are actively involved with projects and specialized programmes, it would be really useful if they could get involved in the whole process of change. Sadly, however, it goes against their mandate.

In the larger monetary picture on health care, one needs to go beyond just figures of how much is spent, and look at how it is spent. A study of eleven states across India has shown that budget allocations to primary health have declined by 2 per cent from the 1980s to the late 1990s (that is from 38 per cent to 36 per cent) (Seetha Prabhu and Selvaraju, 2001). Tertiary services now take up around 22 per cent of the budget, as against 17 per cent in 1985–86. It is obvious that more specialized medical care is taking up a big chunk of the funding, and this in turn is affecting basic care. Yet, there is a limit to which financial inadequacy can be responsible for the malaise that the health-care sector is suffering from. There are other very important reasons why this crucial sector is languishing, and not the least of them is a significant fall in the motivational spirit that once used to drive the medical profession.

All these varied, complex factors—in a diversity of conditions—have led to a collapse in systems, in the quality of medical service to ordinary people, and in the whole journey from ill health to well-being. In the wake of this collapse has come the unprecedented growth of private sector health-care institutions: from the thoroughly unregulated living-room operation theatres to large, corporate hospitals that can ruin many people financially (see Chapter 5). And, if something goes wrong in a healing experience, the ruin can be much more than just financial.

The health system will increasingly need to look at the

prevention and management of chronic, non-communicable lifestyle diseases. The MHFW needs competent, specialized officers who can awaken the sleeping Goliath. Among the many reasons behind the current disarray in which the health scenario finds itself, is the all-important condition of public health institutions and professional capacities. According to Ravi Duggal of CEHAT, Mumbai, the real concerns are: very low health expenditure, three-fourths of which is on salaries; and declining state support for health. The unregulated functioning of the private sector is a major factor, so is the fact that the overall health infrastructure, with the exception of doctors and medicines, has remained very primitive, especially in rural areas. Medical education is heavily subsidized, but 80 per cent of the doctors go in for private practice, laying to waste the huge investment made by the government. Then there is the problem of lack of accountability. The Indian system also lacks a drive for change, or should one say an ability to work on lessons learnt from past experiences? Time and again, especially when disaster strikes, whether it was the plague or the Bhuj earthquake in Gujarat, or rail accidents across the country, the same old problems emerge and there is hardly any wisdom brought to the fresh incident from the past one.

But again, there are some people who make history and their good work makes you wonder why they are such flashes in the pan. When the plague surprised the country with its rather vengeful comeback in 1994, Surat, as any other city, was caught in deep slumber. S.R. Rao couldn't have guessed what it would mean for him. This bureaucrat was sent to post-plague Surat as commissioner some months after the epidemic had visited, struck and gone. Rao got to work on small details like getting open-drains cleaned and covered, tackling housewives who persisted in throwing their daily domestic garbage out of the window on to the roads, and working on the tenacious rodent population of the diamond city. His formula for success was so simple and straightforward that it made one ask, why didn't any other officer do the same? But Rao is a modest man. He believes that there are many motivated bureaucrats in the administrative services whose work remains unsung. The fact is that if there is motivation and drive, problems and hurdles can easily be overcome. The Rao-factor in post-plague Surat is an example of how things can work, how dormant systems can be shaken up to deliver.

The Slumber Breaks, Sometimes

The sleeping Goliath has been stirring for some time now and it is vital to understand that India's achievements, against many odds, have not been small. Life expectancy has climbed from 54 in 1981 to 64.6 in 2000. The crude birth rate is 26.1 (2000) as against 33.9 in 1981. At least 57.3 in every 10,000 suffered from leprosy back in 1981, but now that figure stands at around 3.74. Guineaworm cases were close to 40,000 and the disease has since been eradicated. Polio cases were 29,709, but down to just 265 in 2001. The number of dispensaries and hospitals has almost doubled in two decades, so has the number of doctors. But again, averages mean little in India, where each state is almost like a mini-country, given its population, diverse cultural patterns, and differences in literacy and socio-economic status. If the average IMR is 70, it is 14 in Kerala and 97 in Orissa. If there are 94.9 per 1000 children under 5 years of age who die across India, the figure for the same is 18.8 in Kerala and 137.6 in Madhya Pradesh. Population below the poverty line is 26.1 per cent on an average, but 12.72 in Kerala and 47.15 in

Orissa (*NHP, 2002*). Superimposed on these differences are the variations in socio-economic disparities across states. So what does one do in such a scenario? Well, grab at the rainbows, however small, however fleeting, however feeble. Across the country and the world, India's successes—measured through popular indicators—have been projected. Indians live longer today, fewer children die. According to the Director General of Health Services, infant mortality has declined from 146 per 1000 live births in 1951 to 72 in 1997 and 69 in 2000. In 1951 at least 236 children under the age of 5 used to die for every 1000 births. Today, the figure is 111 children for every 1000 live births. Life expectancy has gone up from 36 years to 62 and in states like Kerala life expectancy is higher than in Washington, DC (World Bank, 2001). The government has taken some forward-looking decisions in the past few years, such as blood safety, a ban on sex determination of unborn babies, on smoking in public places, and on the trade in embryos, to mention a few (see Chapter 9).

But the problem is implementing these decisions, getting the paper tiger to not just roar but also move in for the kill. Many abortions are still being influenced by sex determination tests. In cities like Delhi, it is common to see people smoking under 'No Smoking' signs. This open disregard for governmental guidelines has provoked many experts to suggest that hefty fines be levied on those who violate bans and break rules. Contributing to this lawlessness is illiteracy. After all, in a country where 35 per cent of the population is officially illiterate, an enlightened pursuance of the law cannot possibly be easy. But that is not to be read as something that is impossible to achieve. Considering the intimate link between education, bread-earning capacity and good health, there is little doubt that a large part of the waking-up process will have to be in the spread of literacy or, more importantly, in awareness and knowledge. An issue often considered is whether health and education should be part of the same ministry. With roughly 330 million people who cannot read or write (60 per cent of women and 36 per cent of men), the lack of literacy and education is the basic malaise affecting any good health system. This enormous, unaware population is not just having too many babies, it is also unable to make intelligent choices when it comes to general health—from the need for contraception to consuming the right drugs at the right time, to concocting a home-made oral rehydration solution for a dehydrated baby. The government plans to beef up its Information, Education and Communication (IEC) programme vis-à-vis health but that, pitched against this large, illiterate population, is easier said than done. There is also the other side of illiteracy and socio-economic status—an inability (one cannot but wonder whether it is sometimes just a lack of desire) to question the system and to demand the best of services. According to the NHP of 2002, the present strategy of the MHFW towards spreading information, educating the public and communicating the right messages is not holistic, does not address the real needs of the target population, and relies too heavily on the mass media. The government now wants to target school and college students to spread the message of preventive health care.

The real signs of hope come from actual experiments and programmes that have been done and carried through despite all these hurdles and have shown results. Chapter 9 presents a magnified view of some of these success stories, and admittedly, it has not been easy. With a rapidly growing population and a generally low standard of living, every programme implemented, every reform brought in, has been a complex process with more downs than ups. Added to this is the fact that globalization has come very rapidly to India

(WHO, 2000), and along with it a total flux in the economic situation. These economic changes have not had a positive impact on health scenarios the world over. In fact, India has co-sufferers in other developing nations of Southeast Asia, but the country's population, cultural diversity and size make its problems unique.

Meanwhile, it is almost as though the new NHP of 2002 hopes to do what could not be done in a little less than six decades (For further information see Box: Targeted Goals, p. 97). Despite progressive health indices in some areas, the policy admits that morbidity and mortality levels are still very high in the country, and also links these levels to failures of the public health system at different levels of its functioning. The problem is that the rainbows are too fleeting. They arch over a deeply troubled sector plagued by the three basic issues discussed in this chapter— mismanagement of the sector, roadblocks to implementation of forward-looking policies without delay, and budgetary constraints. It might be said that the order of importance of these three issues is totally open to argument, and can vary depending on who is doing the talking. Government officials will always stress that it is a dearth of finances that has brought health care to its dismal milestone today. Activists and NGOs believe it is a little of each, but would really back the mismanagement theory, while the ordinary user of health services may not be able to analyse the relative importance of any of these factors. Many health ministers and senior government health officials have admitted at public forums that hospital-based health care in cities is becoming the norm and that there is no real practice of public health either by the government or by the general public. For the government and the country's health infrastructure, it is a long road ahead. In earlier years, and in the history of public health, the thrust was on sanitation measures to keep public health problems at bay. The idea was to keep environmental and lifestyle factors in check so that public health problems would not crop up. But somewhere along the way, as microbes were discovered and the means to tackle them found, the concept of treatment became the norm. The privileged who could buy services became distinct from the poor who could not, and the city dweller and the villager became poles apart. Good health came to be looked upon as something to be provided by doctors and hospitals, not something one could achieve by changing one's lifestyle or ensuring environmental cleanliness.

Meanwhile, the desperate demand for good and specialized health services is growing all the time: from Orissa's cyclones to earthquakes in Latur, Bhuj and Garhwal, or in day-to-day routine scenarios, there is a need for quality care, as also timely and targeted intervention. For instance, recent figures show that although less than 20 per cent of the population does not have access to an improved water source, water-borne diseases continue to be a major health hazard (World Bank, 2001). What this implies is that there isn't enough potable water to go around. Something as basic as sanitation facilities are available only to 16 per cent of the population. It is time to break away from confining circumstances and do what is best for the country. If the new health policy hopes to put in place mechanisms to police this anarchic jungle, nothing like it. But the time for implementation is now. It is no longer sufficient for the government to point to all its printed policies and documents and 'successful' programmes and say they've been there, and done it all. The MHFW will need to clearly spell out the policing agency and get a full and functional regulatory order in place. The government, the citizen, institutions and industry must all shoulder responsibility for the condition in which health-care infrastructure finds itself today. Sadly, the average Indian, who is the consumer of these services, has also aided and abetted this downward spiral by never questioning the low quality of health care provided. But, just as the government public health machinery cranks up, the question hour may be on us.

LIST OF RECOMMENDATIONS
(Condensed from Peters et al., 2002)

Bhore Committee, 1946
- No individual should lack access to medical care because of inability to pay for it
- 15 per cent of government expenditure to be devoted to health care

Mudaliar Committee, 1961
- Central government to control communicable diseases
- Strengthen primary health centres

Jain Committee, 1966
- Enhance maternity facilities at each level
- Health insurance for a larger population coverage

Kartar Singh Committee, 1974
- One health supervisor for every four health workers
- Integration of all health programmes and health workers: retrain health workers as multipurpose workers

Srivastava Committee, 1975
- One additional doctor and nurse at PHCs for maternal and child health services
- Establish medical and health education commission

Indian Council of Medical Research—Indian Council for Social Science Research Joint Panel, 1980
- One thirty-bed community health centre per 100,000 population with six general doctors and three specialists
- No further expansion of medical education and drug production but only their rationalization and reorientation

National Health Policy, 1983
- Involvement of private practitioners and NGOs to expand coverage of and access to services
- Establish a nationwide chain of epidemiological stations

TARGETED GOALS
National Health Policy, 2002

(Here is a roadmap for the future, but the point is, is anybody planning to open and follow it, or is it just a sheaf of papers to be buried in a file in some dusty corner of a minister's office?)

2005: Eradicate polio and yaws, eliminate leprosy, establish a system of surveillance, national health accounts and health statistics, increase state health spending from 5.5 to 7 per cent of the budget.

2007: Achieve zero-level growth in HIV/AIDS.

2010: Eliminate kala azar, halve the mortality from TB, malaria and other vector- and water-borne diseases, reduce the prevalence of blindness to 0.5 per cent, IMR to 30 in 1000 and MMR to 100 per 100,000. Reduce the proportion of low birthweight babies to 10 per cent from the current 30 per cent. Utilization of public health facilities to increase from 20 per cent to 75 per cent. Increase health spending from 0.9 per cent of GDP to 2 per cent.

2015: Eliminate lymphatic filariasis.

Sick and Up against a Wall

It is the practices and values accepted in society that raise fundamental ethical issues in medical practice. A doctor relieves pain and cures illness of the patients. He therefore renders a service, which is perhaps the most humane service. At the same time, a doctor cannot afford to be only serving humanity. As a professional he has also to earn his livelihood. When we are looking at the administrators of medical services, we also look at the issue of the financial resources needed for running good public health systems. The point arises whether there should be a commercial approach or a humanitarian approach. How to retain the basic humanitarian approach needed for medical services without at the same time losing sight of the commercial aspects is an issue that must be faced squarely.

—N. Vittal, former Central Vigilance Commissioner, Government of India. Talk delivered at the sixth anniversary meeting of the Medically Aware and Responsible Citizens of Hyderabad, September 2001

Over the past few decades India has witnessed a strange new revolution in the health sector. Strange because although, like all revolutions, it has brought about a plethora of changes, not all the changes have always improved existing conditions. As highlighted in Chapter 4, faced with a crumbling public health infrastructure people have perforce had to seek medical help from the private medical practitioner—the private clinic and hospital. The private practitioner is not a new phenomenon in India; after all, traditional Indian systems of health care have always been provided by this sector, be it the vaidya or the hakim. But the difference is that choosing to visit a private practitioner did not come with the added baggage of a drain on financial resources. Now, the private sector is an expensive health option by any standard. While many of these institutions are trying to make a positive impact by offering the best and most advanced care possible, many more are based on unethical, unregulated and costly medical practice. Across India, there are countless individuals and institutions making money by offering medical services that are nowhere close to what is promised in the Hippocratic Oath, and this is the kind of service that is almost instilling in people a fear of the doctor or the standard health-care institution. It is a mortal fear of falling sick and having to be admitted to a hospital.

O.P. Sharma has known this fear up close. A real estate dealer who lives and works in northwest Delhi, Sharma's seven-year-old son Prakhar has a scarred stump where his right hand should have been, and a badly burnt, contorted face. Prakhar was a normal baby when he was born in 1996 at a private nursing home run out of a residential apartment. While the consultant gynaecologist packed her bags and left for the day as soon as the baby was out of his mother's protective womb, a callous nurse left Prakhar alone in a room, next to an open, electric heater, completely unattended. After sometime, Prakhar's father heard his child wailing continuously, and requested the nurse to let him see the baby.

Though she protested initially, she had to let him in, and Sharma witnessed a scene that would change the course of his life forever, and more so the life of his precious son. His baby had suffered extensive burn injuries from the heater that had been kept too close to him. After the first few days of emergency treatment, Sharma faced the terrible truth: his son would be maimed forever. While cosmetic surgery has brought some shape back to his face, the fingers of the right hand, amputated within a few days of his birth to avoid sepsis, will never be restored (Thapa and Menon, 2000).

Today, looking back, Sharma thinks he made a mistake by going to a small, private clinic. It took his family almost five years to receive the meagre compensation that the consumer court settled for them in a case of medical negligence against the owners of the nursing home. 'No money can really make any difference to my son's life, but I knew I had to do something. I couldn't have taken it lying down,' says Sharma. What drove Sharma through the years was not the money he would receive as compensation, but the relentless force within him to seek justice for his wronged baby.

Sharma has, since then, been able to transcend his own personal loss, grief and anguish, and that of his family's, to speak up and share his painful experience with the media. In other words, he has done everything he could to spread his message. But the larger malaise in the health-care system exists in silence, with numerous such instances that never get discussed or debated. For countless Indians Sharma's would be the tough approach for a variety of reasons. Most importantly, a doctor is almost like God to a patient, and to family and friends of the sick, a person not to be questioned or displeased in any way. This is the reason for the general resignation with which most people accept a doctor's diagnosis, approach and method. Sadly enough, they remain resigned even if something goes terribly wrong in the treatment of the patient. The other important reason why people adopt a path of least resistance is the fact that options for medical care are few.

As highlighted in the previous chapter, the public health system is almost non-existent in many places and the private 'living-room' approach is the most accessible, with its façade of efficiency and plushness. The endless queues one has to face at public sector health institutions compared to the quick appointments with the doctor at private clinics; the frustration of watching the influential and powerful not just jump the queue but also grab beds in well-established public sector hospitals; the inadequacy of medical advice simply because doctors in many public institutions are overworked and short of time to handle the burgeoning out-patient departments; and the derelict condition of neighbourhood government dispensaries that could otherwise have been the best solution are some of the reasons why people end up in private clinics, and are then confronted by commercialized, unethical practices.

In the Service of Humanity?

'Professional medical ethics in the health sector is an area which has not received much attention. Professional practices are perceived to be grossly commercial and the medical profession has lost its elevated position as a provider of basic services to fellow human beings' (*NHP, 2002*). The MCI is supposed to examine complaints of medical malpractice through an internal ethical committee, and possible action can include revoking the registration of the concerned doctor. But it is a power that the MCI has not exercised fully. This lack of action is certainly not because there is no malpractice in India, but because of a nexus that exists between such regulatory agencies and medical professionals—a relationship fuelled by indifference and a lack of concern for the ordinary citizen.

When K.S. Ahluwalia, a professional based in Delhi, took his two-and-a-half-year-old son, Harjot, to a prestigious private hospital in a posh south Delhi locality back in 1993 to have his persistent fever checked, he didn't know he was climbing on to a traumatic roller-coaster ride. Diagnosed as a case of typhoid, Harjot's doctor scribbled the name of an anti-typhoid drug on the prescription chart. The nurse who was to administer the drug injected a strong anti-malarial drug instead. The child suffered a sudden cardiac arrest and although the heart was revived, a lack of efficiency on the part of the hospital staff led to a delay in administering oxygen, and little Harjot suffered permanent brain damage. The perky little boy of the Ahluwalia household had taken a sharp turn on the road of life, and lives on, totally transformed. This led the Ahluwalias first to the gurdwara in search of solace, of solutions, but finally, they found themselves in court, fighting for justice. They won the case against the hospital after a four-year struggle, and today, Ahluwalia views his son's experience as a sacrifice for something worthwhile—dragging unwilling medical professionals towards accountability and responsibility for their actions. That said, Ahluwalia, for obvious reasons, does not believe that the medical profession is dictated by the stringent ethics of serving the sick.

As it turns out, there are countless nursing homes like the one in which Prakhar was born, and where Harjot lost forever his chance to lead a normal life at the tender age of two, at the hands of inadequately trained nurses and because of a general lack of efficient infrastructure. The overarching weakness of these nursing homes is that they are run by unethical doctors who care only about short-term monetary rewards. The last decade of the twentieth century did see some measures taken by the government to try and set right this hopeless situation. In fact, when Harjot suffered this painful and lasting experience, the Consumer Protection Act was not designed to include medical practitioners, a decision that was taken only in the mid-1990s. Soon after this decision was taken by the government, there were serious protests from various medical bodies, all alluding to one issue: the consumer dragnet would stifle and kill the noble and abiding relationship that exists between the doctor and the patient. Meanwhile, for obvious reasons, ordinary citizens across India are fully aware of the fact that in nine cases out of ten there is no such relationship anymore. The general family physician who would venture out at odd hours to attend to a distress call is today a rare species, and experiences like those of the Sharma and Ahluwalia families have put to test the sacred doctor–patient relationship.

The extent of erosion in the ethical foundations of medical practice is also borne out by the enormous growth of quackery across India. While many argue that quacks exist because there is such a pressing need for medical help, the reality is that they owe their existence—and self-taught profession— to a deeply entrenched lack of ethics in medical practice and a total lack of regulation of the sector. Once in a while proactive officers or some other minor circumstance shake up this erosion and laxity. For some time after that there is social debate, government action and some progress. Some years ago, when the Delhi police raided a quack's clinic in west Delhi, he told them he had been a clerk in a prominent city hospital for many years. N.C. Chawla (Menon, 1997) had watched carefully and quietly for so long that he felt confident he could do it himself. What's in a prescription anyway? He slowly moved on in life, opened a 'shop' to treat poor patients, and provided the community with the cheap health-care option they had been searching for. And a quack was born. For twenty-five years, Chawla treated patients for all ailments, and even when he was arrested, residents said, 'He isn't a bad man, in fact his medicines work fine.'

There are no definite figures, but the city of Delhi alone has at least 30,000 quacks according to a recent estimate. The journey towards becoming a quack is almost always catalysed by monetary benefits. Chawla was never really satisfied with the money he earned as a clerk in the hospital where he worked and was always aspiring for bigger things. Except that he believed in the classic short-cut to success. Just watching the doctors around him, Chawla picked up the tricks of the trade, or so he believed. Practising casual medicine is easier in India than in many other countries because of slack laws and a complex mix of systems of medicine, many of which do not require formal training. The traditional neem-hakim who sits at the corner of the street and professes to cure all ailments from a fractured bone to insanity is a living example of how traditional systems of medicine are practised. And yet, it is important to recognize the very significant difference between learned, qualified people who practise traditional systems of medicine and quacks. Quackery is a non-cognizable offence in India. T.A. Majeed should know that. This quack made so much money from people who poured in from all parts of the country for his miracle cure for AIDS that he could afford to live in a three-storeyed mansion called 'Virus', that is set in 34,000 square feet of land in Kochi, Kerala. He came back into public memory recently when his most high-profile case, Chitra, died suffering and unsung in 2001. She battled the disease for many years as it spread through her. But Majeed's wonder drug, Immuno QR, now de-licensed, couldn't possibly have worked. It is well known that AIDS has no real cure yet. But quacks will have you believe anything. Today, Majeed, who is by training a mining engineer, has been barred from manufacturing, producing or advertising any drugs claiming to have anti-HIV properties. This was done through an order of the Supreme Court in early 2002.

But the large majority of quacks continue their practice with no hurdles mainly because their treatment is inexpensive and also readily available. There is also a tangible indifference right across sectors—both public and private—that adds to the 'fear' dimension. According to a media report of an incident that occurred at the Sadvichar Eye Hospital in Ahmedabad, Gujarat in July 2001 (*Indian Express,* 2001), thirty-eight people were partially blinded due to callously executed cataract surgery. Three people lost both their eyes, seven lost one, and twenty-eight developed complications that could lead to blindness in the near future. A week after surgery, when bandages were removed, all these people had already developed infections. The hospital, run by a trust, dismissed its own moral responsbility, saying that it was a solution used during surgery that caused the trouble. The solution is used to clean the cataract before excising it, and also after surgery. But the incredible part of this story is not just the total carelessness with which the procedure was carried out, but also the way in which responsibility was shrugged off after the mishap.

The urgent need to implement laws that can ensure the ethical practice of medicine is being felt across the country today, and in all sectors that offer medical services. This has become significant because of the large number of people who now rely on private health-care service providers. The ethics of medical practice, the cost of health care, and the overall regulation of systems become more challenging when it comes to the private sector, and the government is currently in the process of developing mechanisms that can begin to address this lacuna in the overall functioning of the health-care system—public or private.

Public or Private, What's the Choice?

The Escorts Heart Institute and Research Centre (EHIRC), although a typical private institution where a substantial amount of money is required to undergo any procedure, is run with amazing efficiency and scores of heart surgeries—major and minor—are performed each day by a strong and ever-growing team of doctors. Dr Naresh Trehan, the cardiac surgeon who is behind the genesis of the EHIRC, has also kept his promise to the country in the sense that the most modern techniques are used and patients are assured of the best possible surgery, treatment and post-surgical care. Using a tested, well-lubricated hospital administrative system, this large, corporate hospital is run with almost text-book efficiency. The EHIRC, while offering private health care not every Indian can afford, has maintained high ethical standards in the treatment of heart patients from all over India and the subcontinent.

Efficiency, single-window jobs, quick results are the magic words that have attracted people towards private care, and data from the National Sample Survey Organization (NSSO) have shown clear evidence of a decline in the overall use of public health care. From the mid-1980s to the mid-1990s there was a 3 per cent decline in the share of public institutions providing out-patient services in rural areas, and a 5 per cent decline in urban areas (Duggal, 2001). According to the NHP of 2002, of all the people who seek out-patient department services in the country, less than 20 per cent visit public hospitals, and of those who need in-patient care, less than 45 per cent avail of the services in a public institution.

Taking in-patient care as an example, public institutional contribution came down by 40 per cent in urban areas over a ten-year period from 1986 to 1996 (Duggal, 2001). Duggal says: 'Public health services have become synonymous with preventive and promotive care, and three-fourths of all such services are from the public health system, while the private system, for all the obvious reasons, has had a negligible role to play.' Ambulatory care is often provided by the private sector (more than 80 per cent). Such private care is particularly common in Punjab, Haryana, Uttar Pradesh, Maharashtra, West Bengal and Bihar. Again, within the private sector, it is the individual practitioner who hogs some 70 per cent of the share, whereas hospitals take upto 23 per cent. For in-patient care, the share of the private sector in hospitalizations has gone up by 33 per cent from the 1980s to the 1990s. Duggal has also found that for all social and economic classes, the private doctor is the biggest provider of out-patient care. Amazingly, the top 20 per cent expenditure class is also the biggest user of public hospital conveniences. This is ruining health security for the millions.

Analyses of the 42nd and 52nd rounds of the *National Sample Survey* (*NSS*) show how more and more people are now using the private sector for health care and medical needs (Baru, 2001). Of course, the growth of the private sector is varied across states. For instance, Baru's analysis of the 42nd NSS found that Andhra Pradesh, Gujarat, Maharashtra, Kerala and Punjab have a higher private-bed strength than the public sector. In some of the poorer states, the public sector is used much more. These statistics may be interpreted as a healthy growth in private health care, but the disturbing fact is that few Indians can afford it, and often make out-of-pocket payments for the same by compromising on many other basic needs, even nutrition.

Can Indians Afford Sickness?

On the whole, Indians cannot afford sickness at all. It is this lack of affordability that adds to the fear of ending up in a hospital or having to depend more than usual on a doctor or medical institution. Almost 90 per cent of Indian families earn their living by working in the informal sector and have almost no protection against death and disease: 'no health care benefits, paid sick leave, maternity benefits, insurance or old age pension' (Gumber and Kulkarni, 2001). Gumber and Kulkarni argue that while terrible poverty and sickness push the poor into a trap, they end up spending more on health than people who are financially better off. It is a double whammy for them—the disease stalks them and becomes a sponge on their meagre earnings, and they get no wages when they are sick, which further weakens them financially and mentally. Apparently, only 9 per cent of the Indian workforce is covered by some form of medical insurance. This figure is low because of the government's emphasis on free care, but the problem is that free care is really not free. Although the informal sector contributes significantly to the economy, the people who fall into this section of society are not covered by any health benefits, get no paid sick-leave, or maternity benefits.

At least a quarter of our population lives below the poverty line and cannot afford to pay for health care (Seetha Prabhu and Selvaraju, 2001). The most serious flip side of such urban care is that a substantial 23.6 per cent of urban Indians also subsist below the poverty line. Adding to the burden that the less privileged carry is the fact that the rich always misuse government support. It is indeed ironical, as a recent study by the National Council for Applied Economic Research (NCAER) has shown, that India's richest 20 per cent have the luxury of using three times as much government subsidy on health as the poorest 20 per cent of the population. According to the World Bank, more than half the total annual expenditure by an average Indian is on health care (World Bank, 2001). Therefore, of all the people who are hospitalized at any one time, more than 40 per cent borrow money or liquidize assets to pay medical bills. Each year, at least 2.2 per cent of the population drops below the poverty line simply because of exorbitant medical bills paid out of their pockets.

It is not surprising then that health and well-being are being defined by each individual's socio-economic reach, rather than by his or her actual need for health services. Making this economic gap worse is the fact that public health care has not really remained the cheap alternative it was always professed to be. Although it is inexpensive when compared with private care, public health care has also become more and more costly over the years. Baru's analysis has shown that between 1986 and 1996 the cost of public sector hospitalization in urban areas actually went up by 470 per cent, and by 343 per cent in the private sector. The escalating cost of consumables is a significant reason for this increase in the cost of public health care. In the last few years, the middle class has moved from public to private health care, and this has impacted on the quality of health care provided by the public sector. The cost of in-patient care grew at 26–31 per cent annually, and out-patient care costs grew at the rate of about 15–16 per cent between 1986–87 and 1995–96 (Gumber and Kulkarni, 2001).

More than 80 per cent of all health spending by Indians is

on the private sector, and this is supposed to be one of the highest proportions in the world (Peters et al., 2002). As a result, the World Bank study found that,

> poorer households purchase less curative health care from the private sector than do richer households. Partly because of inability to pay and the lack of risk pooling, the poor are much less likely to be hospitalized. Across India, those above the poverty line have more than double the hospitalization rates of the poor. (World Bank, 2001)

A major hurdle in the regulation of health financing is the fact that just about 10 per cent of the population has any form of insurance against disease and debilitation. As a result, if a single family member is hospitalized even once, the whole family can face complete financial ruin, however temporary. More than half of a hospitalized Indian's average annual expenditure is on health care, and more than 40 per cent of people who need to be admitted to a hospital have to either borrow money to cover these expenses or sell their assets (Peters et al., 2002). This total erosion of financial stability can be so complete that an ordinary person who could afford a decent living can come back from hospital impoverished. In fact, according to the NSSO, this happened to about a quarter of the population in 1996. While the medical insurance sector has recently seen some reform, it still remains out of reach for most people, as do good doctors whom people can trust their lives with.

A Scarcity of Good Doctors

There are more than 500,000 registered medical practitioners in India, of whom more than 400,000 are allopathic doctors

(*Economic Survey, 1999–2000*). Hardly a quarter of all the doctors in the country are prepared to serve in remote areas where their services are most needed. This is a gap that is deeply felt, often with very serious consequences, but even the government is struggling to find ways and means to overcome this problem. If one were to stop and look at the kind of health-care facilities that are available to different sections of society, there would be tangible evidence of this inequality. The NHP of 2002 has found that, while the average IMR in India is 70 per 1000, it is 83 for scheduled castes and 84.2 for scheduled tribes. While on an average 94.9 children below the age of 5 die per 1000 live births, the same figure is 119.3 and 126.6 for scheduled castes and tribes, respectively. On an average, 47 per cent of all children are underweight, of which 53.5 per cent and 55.9 per cent are for scheduled castes and tribes, respectively. But the number of doctors actually at hand to treat these less privileged is few and many of them never really report on duty in less-known parts of the country (see Chapter 8).

The scarcity of doctors is compounded by a shortfall in the infrastructural network. The National Population Policy (NPP) of 2000 had put forward an estimate of shortage: 1513 PHCs, 23,190 sub-primary centres, and 2899 CHCs. There is also an incredible shortage of staff—1525 physicians, 1774 paediatricians, and 6635 specialists. Most doctors (85 per cent)—qualified and unqualified—are in the private sector. The NHP of 2002 plans to address the problem of inequitable distribution of medical staff between urban and rural areas, as well as within the more- and less-privileged parts of urban areas. The policy says:

No incentive system attempted so far has induced private medical personnel to go to such areas; and, even in the public health sector, the effort to deploy medical personnel in such under-served areas, has usually been a losing battle. In such a situation, the possibility needs to be examined of entrusting some limited public health functions to nurses, paramedics and other personnel from the extended health structure after imparting adequate training to them. (*NHP, 2002*)

Along with the shortage of medical and paramedical staff in sheer numbers, there is also a question of quality. Medical education across the country is 'highly uneven and in several instances even sub-standard,' according to the *NHP, 2002*. Medical science has grown more than any other discipline in the last few years, but its syllabi have remained, in large measure, insulated from change; the doctors too are often unaware of the latest changes in the world of medicine. The NHP of 2002 hopes to come up with serious recommendations to revise the curricula to fill this void. This is in realization of the fact that medical education in the country is today uncontrolled and sub-standard. There are many colleges that have grown out of nothing, and permissions to open a medical college are not much of a challenge anymore. There are colleges which have only a building and equipment, but no affiliation to a hospital where students can get practical training. Capitation fees and donations are now quite common for admission to medical colleges, just as it is with other professional courses. However, few realize that medical education is different from all other kinds of education, and that since a medical student is being trained and taught to save human lives, he must be taught to do it in the best way and through as ethical and honest a route as possible.

It is Time to Regulate the Private Sector

According to the *NSS* (52nd round), 82 per cent of out-patient department care and 56 per cent of in-patient care is provided by the private sector (Seetha Prabhu and Selvaraju, 2001). Against these facts it is ironical that there is no real system of regulation of private sector hospitals. The MHFW clearly states that it can do nothing about the many pitfalls of private health care, simply because the policy doesn't allow it. Perhaps it is time for reconsideration, because this particular private service can stand between life and death for many people. The process of reform, in all fairness, has begun. With unusual alacrity, the NHP of 2002 has stated that instead of trying to debate whether private care is good or bad, it is better to accept it as a reality that cannot be wished away. Meanwhile, what the government does want to do is to establish a clear-cut regulatory mechanism for the private health-care sector so as to monitor the adherence to minimum standards of medical care in private hospitals, nursing homes and diagnostic centres. The same applies to doctors who practise privately. The dearth of rules and regulations has created what experts would like to call anarchy. The fact that the private sector has grown to provide health care with little policing is a global phenomenon. According to *The World Health Report*:

> In India, mechanisms for monitoring, let alone regulating, the private sector have not kept pace with its expansion, despite concerns about quality of care. Health professionals are aware of practice-related laws but know that enforcement is weak or non-existent and that professional associations, which are nominally responsible for self-regulation, are also ineffective. (WHO, 2000)

There is also the rampant and unfortunate culture of the public sector subsidizing private practice, with physicians often working for the public sector also indulging in private practice for the extra money. This kind of moonlighting proves very expensive for the health system.

The NHP of 2002 clearly admits that owing to a general decadence, the country's government hospitals are quickly reaching a state of total disrepair. There are not enough doctors and paramedical staff, equipment is ancient and often unusable, essential drugs are often unavailable, administration is a nightmare, and overall facilities and maintenance are in a shambles. As mentioned earlier in the chapter, this has driven many people to private hospitals, but the sad part is that this has been with a lot of reluctance on their part. Private care is the tougher, more distant option, considering that at least a fourth of the country lives below the poverty line. But people still try to avoid the abyss that a government hospital has begun to represent, and prefer paying for private health care by compromising on things as basic as daily food and nutrition.

Much of this change has been wrought by an erosion of ethical practices of medicine, and this has in turn been fuelled by an over-riding concern for monetary rewards. Supporting this preoccupation of the average doctor is the qualitative decline of the less-expensive public sector and the consequent mushrooming of the private sector. It has now emerged as a really complex problem, with no easy solutions. Again, a lot of the solutions will have to come from the people themselves—just as Sharma and Ahluwalia went in search of solutions. Except that, in their case, it was after so much trauma and loss.

The public remains uninformed about much of the health system. It knows little about whether health services are appropriate, who is benefiting from them, whether quality is sufficient, or whether people are getting good value from public and private spending on health. Equity, quality and accountability are badly wanting in both the public and private health sectors. (Peters et al., 2002)

In the past few years there has been some effort at creating legal procedures that allow ordinary people redressal against the backlash of a lack of motivation, but it is still a reality most patients are faced with. Meanwhile, it is also intriguing that programmes like immunization and contraceptive services have seen very little investment from the private sector. It is actively involved with antenatal care and obstetric services, perhaps because it is such a lucrative business, considering India's high birth rate. These are the worries that individuals have when it comes to private health care—the priorities seem totally lopsided, and money becomes central to the whole process of healing.

The Drug Makers

India has one of the most developed drug industries in the Third World and is capable of self-reliance in the production of most drugs. In the light of this, it is ironical that it has not been able to rationalize its drug policy and ensure availability of essential and life-saving drugs to the large, vulnerable section of its population that needs them the most.

—VHAI, 1997

One of the developing world's most advanced drug industries finds itself at the crossroads today. Having grown in an almost boundless fashion for many decades based on the freedom provided by the Indian Patent Act of 1970, the Indian pharmaceutical industry is now bracing itself for fresh regulations from the World Trade Organization (WTO), which are to be clamped very soon in 2005. For an industry that has persistently tinkered with formulations originally created in the industrialized world and marketed them in cheaper and more accessible forms, there is now pressure to innovate and create novel drug designs. Whether it is ethical or unethical to do what the Indian pharmaceutical industry did all these years, the jury remains out on that question. But it did change the whole scenario of drug development and availability of life-saving medicines for the people of India, and for people from other countries. In fact, the success of the pharmaceutical industry in redefining prices of drugs was so far-reaching that many other global manufacturers have been forced to reduce their prices of life-saving drugs. Back in the 1960s, Indian drug prices were considered amongst the highest in the world (VHAI, 1997). Imports were the country's mainstay. Then came the Indian Patent Act of 1970 which allowed and recognized the patenting of the 'process' of drug manufacturer, but not the product that was patented. As a result, Western drugs were re-formulated with minor changes and new processes patented—like taking a different route to reach the same destination. This was much simpler than developing a new drug, but in recent years there have been protests, such as the global reaction to cheaper HIV/AIDS antiretroviral drugs developed and sold by the Indian pharmaceutical giant Cipla, from various quarters.

According to the NHP of 2002, India's relatively low-cost health-care system owes a lot to the 'widespread availability of indigenously manufactured drugs and vaccines', but 'there is an apprehension that globalization will lead to an increase in the costs of drugs, thereby leading to rising trends in overall health costs.' In fact, experts feel that the 2005 deadline has already placed pressure on leading Indian pharmaceutical companies, all of whom have now begun serious product research and development in preparedness for the new intellectual property regime. It is, therefore, an industry in the midst of change, some turmoil and serious redefinition of profiles. It is understandable that developing countries like India are preoccupied with the kind of impact the global adoption of intellectual property regimes will have on nationwide public health programmes since it is clear that total patent protection will mean escalation in drug prices besides a squeeze in the choice of drugs available to people across the country (Commission on Intellectual Property Rights, 2002).

Since the WTO came into existence in 1995, and with the birth of Trade Related Aspects of Intellectual Property Rights (TRIPS) making it mandatory for all developing nations to build in laws for twenty-year patent protection for all new products and processes emerging from all technological fields, the pharmaceutical industry being no exception, the impact of such rules on the health of the less privileged has been a matter of controversy and debate worldwide. Again, it is the pharmaceutical industry in the developed countries that has been one of the strongest proponents of a worldwide extension of intellectual property rights. In fact, the Commission on Intellectual Property Rights (2002) highlights how:

> without the incentive of patents it is doubtful the private sector would have invested so much in the discovery or development of medicines, many of which are currently in use both in developed and developing countries. Successive surveys have shown that the pharmaceutical companies, more than any other sector, think patent protection to be very important in maintaining their R&D [research and development] expenditures and technological innovation.

Realizing the fact that the kind of changes the new patent regime under TRIPS demanded would require wide-ranging amendments in national patent laws, it was decided that developing countries with economies in transition could take till January 2005 to do so. Therefore, India's long honeymoon with reverse engineering is drawing to a close.

But it has been a great honeymoon. Within a few years of

new drugs appearing in the market in countries like the USA and in Europe, there were cheaper versions of the same drugs available in vast quantities in India. As a result, not just domestic markets, but exports too, boomed. Now, with TRIPS, prices of drugs are bound to increase. According to the former health secretary J.A. Chowdhury (WHO, 2000), 90 per cent of medicines in the country's central drugs list were simply generic drugs, not patented medications. This indicates that the Indian pharmaceutical industry might do well to pull up its socks, but there is a catch. Experts explain how research in the pharmaceutical industry is ridden with risks, made especially significant because this is a commercial, industrial sector that relies almost totally on its R&D for sustenance (Sheth, 2001). Most drug formulation development is a long-drawn-out process, with success a rarity, and a huge upfront investment both in terms of infrastructure and human resource. Sheth says: 'For every 10,000 New Chemical Entities (NCE) in discovery, ten enter pre-clinical development, five enter human trials and one may be approved. For India, the estimate for the development of a single NCE is often quoted to be US$ 90–100 million' (Sheth, 2001). And yet, experts believe that in the long run, stringent patent laws will strengthen the R&D sector of the Indian pharmaceutical industry. To quote Sir Richard Sykes, former chairman of Glaxo Smith Kline, as writing in the report of the Commission on Intellectual Property Rights (2002):

I do not believe that TRIPS will prevent other developing countries like Brazil and India from obtaining access to the medicines they need. On the other hand, I firmly believe that these countries have the capacity to nurture research-based pharmaceutical industries of their own, as well as other innovative industries, but this will only happen when they provide the intellectual property protection that is enshrined in TRIPS.

All that has been rosy about the Indian pharmaceutical industry will need redefinition when it will have to rise to the challenge of product patents that will come into force in the country from 2005. Here, India is not in a happy situation at all. There are very few companies that have undertaken any serious R&D investments, and they are nowhere on the global scale. According to Professor Ranjit Roy Chaudhury, President of the Delhi Society for Promotion of Rational Use of Drugs (DSPRUD), many pharmaceutical units in India will go out of business by 2005. In India, Ranbaxy, according to Sheth, has built 'strategic initiatives to become a global company', and Reddy's Laboratories has apparently earned most from R&D. In fact, collaborative R&D efforts are becoming an established norm for mainline Indian pharmaceutical companies to be able to take forward state-of-the-art research initiatives. Meanwhile, media reports indicate that the 2003 World Health Assembly (WHA) had agreed to allow countries to compel global pharmaceutical companies to license them patents in case of emergencies.

While the global scene and India's final foothold in the changed scenario will bear itself out in the decade ahead, the more immediate problem for the country is regulation of the drugs industry. The rules and regulations that should, and do on paper, govern the entry and sale of new drugs in the market are obsolete and ineffective, and it is easy to find one's way around the rules. At a time when new molecules are being discovered and marketed at a very fast pace, it is imperative for India's regulatory and administrative system to become more stringent.

Too Many Bosses

In keeping with the common practice of Indian governance, drugs and pharmaceuticals come under multiple ministerial charges—the Ministry of Chemicals and Fertilizers (MCF) and the MHFW. The MCF's mandate is to formulate policy to govern the industry, including regulation and drug pricing. Meanwhile, the MHFW is responsible for quality control of drugs, the development and introduction of new drugs, and the enforcement of quality control and all other necessary regulations. As is quite obvious, the interests and priorities of both these ministries are quite disparate, and that is why the quality of drugs has suffered at the cost of unregulated growth of the industry through thousands of small manufacturing units. This has been in the interest of the MCF. Since the MCF is the nodal ministry for framing the drug policy, decisions regarding production of drugs are not governed as much by their necessity but more by their profit margins. Meanwhile, the Indian government is working on a new drug policy for the country. It is about time, really, because even with a bundle of amendments, the Drugs and Cosmetics Act (DCA) of 1940 is inadequate in today's changed scenario. The J.L. Hathi Committee in 1975 had recommended that 116 essential drugs be produced on a priority basis. It is this committee that had laid down guidelines for the basic administration of the drugs industry till the release of the Drug Policy of 1994. The problem is that the centre and the states are both involved in the various aspects of making drugs available to the people for consumption, and that means chaos. Under the DCA of 1940, the central government is supposed to regulate the import of drugs and approve new drugs. Manufacture, sale and distribution come under the state government and this is what leads to so much variation and lack of rigour in the market.

Can We Rationalize Drug Use?

Driven by a complex system of multiple ministerial controls and the lack of a strong and updated drug policy at the level of the central and the state governments, India has witnessed a rampant growth in the irrational use of medicines in civil society—whether at the level of the individual or of the institution. It has taken action from NGOs and individuals to try and focus attention on the danger of irrational drug use in India (For further information see Box: Making a Difference, pp. 128–29). The WHO has conducted studies in over thirty countries and has found that just by encouraging the rational use of drugs, medication costs are known to drop by a significant 30–40 per cent margin. Even beginning to work towards the rational use of drugs will involve many initiatives, such as, analysis of lists of essential drugs; understanding drug procurement and quality control, a drug pricing mechanism, availability and distribution, and detailed information about drugs; besides, of course, spreading awareness among common people about drug use.

Unfortunately, the Indian pharmaceutical industry has little or no interest in the rational use of drugs. With millions of people falling sick frequently, and several who are too poor and vulnerable to stave off the pressures of an aggressive market, added to which is the lack of a strong rational drug policy, pharmaceutical companies have been doing brisk business. In the late 1990s, VHAI estimated that there were at least 80,000 formulations in the Indian market, and with no system of central registration of such formulations, rational drug use is a pipedream. If a single antibiotic can be available in eighty to a hundred different brands, confusion will naturally follow. This kind of confusion is also increased by the fact that different states work independently to get drugs out in the market. Also, drug packaging doesn't leave much chance for rational use, because statutory warnings or contra-indications, adverse effects and side-effects of drugs are mentioned in such fine print that they can hardly be read (VHAI, 1997).

The Drug Pricing Policy is in some ways lopsided, and makes the production of non-essential drugs more profitable. Meanwhile, producing life-saving, essential drugs is not as viable a business deal. 'The majority of drugs that lie outside the purview of "price control" are precisely those that should not have been marketed at all' and this list is growing all the time (VHAI, 1997). Added to cost is the fact that the maximum allowable post-manufacturing expenses have also grown, which include packing, trade margins and profits. A shrinking price-control basket, along with these factors, has led to an increase in the price of drugs. Thus, while drugs cost less in India than in many developed nations, they are still beyond the reach of the average Indian who often has to make the tough decision of going without certain medicines simply because they are unaffordable. Rationalizing drug use will also mean having to tackle pricing of drugs and drawing up a realistic list of drugs that should remain 'price-controlled'.

Irrational drug use has a lot to do with the way pharmacies have become shops in India. Your friendly, local chemist is friendly, yes, but is he qualified too? Every chemist shop, ideally, should employ a qualified pharmacist. A chemist—who is after all a retailer—will always push the most expensive drug, rather than the most effective one. Such a system makes it impossible for actual health considerations to be the focus in determining drug choice; instead, it is always the market that will define drug choice. The problem of over-the-counter sales of prescription drugs is also a big factor that affects the system. Buying drugs in this casual manner is the best-known and established form of drug purchase in the country. This is a well-established practice that can be changed only if rules are taken seriously and the government decides to implement the many laws it has on paper. Today, a chemist's shop resembles a doctor's clinic, with customers unaware of the drugs they consume on the chemist's advice. What has to be done, at a minimum, is to train pharmacists, make sure that a chemist's shop is not like any other retail shop, ensure that doctors learn more about pharmacology, and that the patient learns to question the incomprehensible, spidery prescription he or she carries straight to the chemist without even a second glance. A general lack of awareness about medicines, a total acceptance of a doctor's prescription with no questions asked about the antibiotics prescribed, the common belief that medication will set everything right are all factors that also add to the irrational approach to medication and drugs.

There is also the worrying matter of medical education and its relevance to this sector. Pharmacology lacks cadres and specialized structures in the profession per se, says Roy Chaudhury. Budding doctors are taught about drugs by using the generic name of the drug. In reality there are thousands of brand names—there can be hundred different brands for the same generic antibiotic, so it isn't just the consumer who is confused, it is also the doctor and the chemist (VHAI, 1997). Studies in India have shown that doctors are not given thorough training on rational drug use or drug selection. Unbelievable though it may sound, much of a doctor's knowledge about drugs and their use comes from medical sales representatives who regularly and persistently go about selling or recommending specific brands of drugs (VHAI, 1997).

Incentives and schemes offered by such representatives are also known to influence prescription patterns.

Quantity, Yes, but Quality?

Good manufacturing practice and quality management systems are just a meaningless string of words for many medicine manufacturers in India who treat their business like any other and at the cost of quality. Considering that medicines can as easily take lives as they can give lives, it is strange that the government—which must obviously be in the know of how indifferently the sector is being handled—is saying or doing little to change the situation. The most common cases of spurious drugs affecting health have occurred through contaminated intravenous fluids and other such common hospital consumables. In 1986, fourteen people succumbed to adulterated glycerol at the J.J. Hospital in Mumbai. According to VHAI, a commission was set up under Justice Bakhtavar Lentin in response to a complaint filed by Dr N.H. Antia, a well-known community health worker. The commission's report says:

> These pages describe and illustrate the ugly facets of the human mind and human nature—misuse of ministerial power and authority; apathy towards human life; corruption; nexus and pro quo between unscrupulous license holders, analytical laboratories, elements in the Industries Department, controlling the awarding of contracts, manufacturers, traders, merchants, suppliers, the Food and Drug Administration (FDA) and persons holding ministerial rank. (VHAI, 1997)

The second schedule of the DCA is supposed to govern

the quality of drugs manufactured and licensed for use in the country. This schedule spells out that the standards of quality enlisted in the Indian pharmacopoeia will apply for all drugs mentioned in it. Interestingly, the pharmacopoeia has been published only four times over the last half century, between 1955 and 2000, with six supplements as updates. In the US, the same is brought out once every five years with an addendum each year (Pabrai, 2001). Says Pabrai:

> The growing complacency towards the inefficiency and corruption in the country has not spared the drug control departments. Stories in this regard are becoming more frequent and sensational than before. The problem needs to be handled with firmness by people who are upright. There is no dearth of them but the fear generated by the drug mafia seems to be preventing them from performing their duties without fear and favour. Necessary encouragement and protection must be provided to such persons. (Pabrai, 2001)

There is another factor that makes the whole system of regulating the medicine market in the country more complex, and this is the fact that there is a plethora of medicinal systems to follow. While allopathy remains the most common choice, there are other streams under the Indian systems of medicine (ISM) such as ayurveda, unani and many more. It would help the average Indian if the many problems of running this highly unorganized sector across the country could be ironed out, and systems put in place. It is, after all, considered a relatively safe, more natural method of medication by many. If subjected to the same rigours of quality control as allopathic medicines, the ISM could fulfil medication needs of several people. There are already millions of people who only consume drugs from the ISM. Roy Chaudhury, who has spent a lifetime working with allopathic drugs, also believes there is need for a strong, complementary system of traditional medicine. And this system too will need to address the issue of quality control in the manufacture of medicines.

Where, then, lie the solutions? Doctors will always remain friends with the pharmaceutical industry—the consumer can only try to rise above it with awareness and more knowledge to be able to question drug choices. If a programme of rational drug use, either at national or state level, can really help in increasing access to good quality medicines, improving the methods of prescribing drugs and pressing for maximization of existing resources there may be change (For further information see Box: Making a Difference, pp. 128–29). India perhaps needs a National Drug Authority (NDA) to step beyond the natural dichotomy that exists between the MCF and the MHFW. What is required is a neat, not necessarily too long, essential drugs list, with separate identities for drugs used at different levels of health care. As VHAI's commission report states:

> Unfortunately, promotion of the drug trade has been associated with unethical marketing practices and violation of ethical criteria drawn up by the WHO. Influence on prescription practices of doctors and the kinds of drugs to be included in the National Health Programmes are well known. A sound Drug Policy ensures the manufacture of essential drugs, withdrawal of irrational and hazardous drugs, provision of unbiased drug information, quality control, reasonable drug prices, technological self-reliance and ethical marketing practices. (VHAI, 1997)

Tall order, but nevertheless a very good place to start.

MAKING A DIFFERENCE

'At nearly every hospital I visited there were complaints that drugs were not available. Other complaints related to the quality of drugs, their procurement and distribution, and the information given to patients about the use of drugs. Each hospital had its own list of drugs, medicines came to hospitals under many brand names, supply was erratic and the prescribing, very often, unrestrained.'

—Dr Harsh Vardhan, former minister for Health and Family Welfare, Government of Delhi (DSPRUD, 1999).

Delhi is the only state in India that actually has a Rational Drug Policy. Now, Maharashtra, Rajasthan, Himachal Pradesh, Punjab, Tamil Nadu and West Bengal are emulating the same. Bihar and Madhya Pradesh have joined the programme (DSPRUD, 1999). It is almost three decades since WHO first introduced the concept of essential drugs and their rational use. Yet, it took the government nearly two decades to get started on this. In 1994, the then Health Minister, Dr Harsh Vardhan, kicked off a programme to promote the rational use of drugs in the National Capital Region. The Government of Delhi, along with DSPRUD, and with assistance from the India WHO Programme in Essential Drugs, managed a partnership of politicians, bureaucracy and professionals to change things for the better.

The Delhi government worked on a new drug policy based on international norms with the help of DSPRUD. In 1994, an essential drugs list was created and training programmes to make professionals aware of the rational use of drugs were conducted. Within a year, there was a centralized, pooled procurement system, a system of quality control and good manufacturing practice, and a set-up to conduct research and monitor drug use. Ethical criteria for the advertisement and promotion of drugs were established in 1996, and by 1997 a State Drugs Formulary was ready. By 1997, drug availability in Delhi's health centres had gone up manifold, pooled procurement meant that the Delhi government was getting drugs at 30 per cent of the cost incurred by other government agencies and, with the phasing out of unnecessary drugs, essential drugs became available on demand.

DSPRUD was started in 1991 as an advisory to Dr Harsh Vardhan and later became a full-fledged society. Now DSPRUD works in collaboration with WHO on essential drugs and the rational use of drugs. Roy Chaudhury's shopping list for success is simple, yet effective: do not use too many drugs; let hospitals have a central pool of drugs, with central purchase mechanisms; maintain a double-envelope system for drugs procurement—technical criteria for the drug in one envelope and the quotation in another, so that only once the technical criteria are met is there a need to open the second envelope; do not recognize any agents; ensure that a manufacturer has a laboratory for quality control; and, of course, provide information to the patient.

In the Global Scheme of Things

> Measured in terms of infant mortality rates, maternal mortality, life expectancy and nutrition, the health of the Indian population has improved dramatically over the past 50 years. Yet, despite these achievements, wide disparities exist between different income groups, between rural and urban communities, between different states and even districts within states, and a big gap from the level attained by high middle income and advanced developed countries.
>
> —*Report of the Committee on India Vision 2020*, Planning Commission, 2002

In June 2000, a committee was set up by the Planning Commission to visualize and construct a vision for the year 2020 for the people of India. More than thirty experts from across the country got together and, after two years of discussion and deliberation, came up with *India Vision 2020*. The basic spirit of this exercise was to reflect on 'unfinished tasks of nation-building and the country's future possibilities' (Planning Commission, 2002). Chaired by Dr S.P. Gupta, member, Planning Commission, this committee has placed on record how the vision document can 'serve to indicate broad lines of policy and strategy by which India can emerge as a far stronger, more prosperous and more equitable nation in the coming years'. But if the current health-sector scenario and India's present position among the nations of the world as regards the status of public health in the country are any indication, then realizing these laudable dreams will be no mean task. In the *HDR, 2003*, India ranked 127 in a grouping of 175 nations, with a Human Development Index (HDI) value of 0.590 against the world average of 0.722. The UNDP's definition of the HDI is a composite index measuring average achievements in three basic dimensions of human development—longevity, knowledge and standard of living. These three dimensions of the HDI are put together and calculated by using the indices of life expectancy at birth, adult literacy rate, and the per capita GDP in purchasing power parity (PPP US$). In other words, the HDI has a lot to do with the health and general well-being of the people of a nation.

This is India's rank when India has a number of standard health indices that seem to chart a path of progress that the country has been on for the last few decades. Most significantly, life expectancy at birth has more than doubled in the last half century. At the time of Independence, life expectancy was, on an average, 30 years. Between 1970 and 1996, the national average grew from 49.7 years to 60.7 years (*National Human Development Report* [*NHDR*], *2001*). The IMR has also declined significantly from 146 per 1000 live births in 1951 to just 70 in the year 2000. The world average for IMR in 2000 was 56 (UNDP, 2002). The government is proud of many of the achievements in the health sector, and the NHP of 2002 underscores the importance of the eradication of small pox and guinea worm disease from the country. Polio is the government's next target, followed by kala azar and leprosy (see Table 1).

Table 1: Health Achievements over Half a Century

Indicator	1951	1981	2000
Demographic Changes			
Life Expectancy	36.7	54.0	64.6
Crude Birth Rate	40.8	33.9	26.1
Crude Death Rate	25.0	12.5	8.7
Infant Mortality Rate	146.0	110.0	70.0
Epidemiological Shifts			
Malaria (cases in millions)	75.0	2.7	2.2
Leprosy (cases per 10,000 population)	57.3	3.74	38.1
Small Pox (No. of cases)	>44,887	Eradicated	Nil
Guinea Worm (No. of cases)	Not recorded	>39,792	Eradicated
Polio	Not recorded	29,709	265
Infrastructure			
SC/PHC/CHC	725	57,363	163,181
Dispensaries and Hospitals (All)	9209	23,555	43,322
Beds (Private and Public)	117,198	569,495	870,161
Doctors (Allopathy)	61,800	2,68,700	503,900
Nursing Personnel	18,054	1,43,887	737,000

Source: *National Health Policy, 2002*, Department of Health, Ministry of Health and Family Welfare, Government of India.

Across the world, indicators of healthy living are critical to defining the success of societies. In fact these indicators have also defined the success of civilizations. These indices are vital to the evaluation of a development process (*NHDR, 2001*). And yet, for India, the composite picture is still one of a country that has much to achieve before reaching global standards. Also, these figures must not be assessed in isolation but against the targets that were set and what other countries have achieved. The problem is that we set our sights too low. The doubling of life expectancy at birth in the last five decades, for instance, does not hold up against advances made in the developing countries of East Asia and Latin America, where life expectancy is the same as in developed nations (*NHDR, 2001*).

Even in the strife-torn neighbouring island-nation of Sri Lanka, life expectancy at birth is 71.6 years, and the IMR is 17 per 1000 live births. More than 90 per cent of Sri Lanka's adult population is literate (UNDP, 2003). The HDI is 0.741, higher than the world average. According to the World Bank, 'Sri Lanka has recorded impressive achievements in health, nutrition, and family planning with relatively low levels of public expenditure on health. A commitment to broader social development including education is a factor in its success.' Fertility is almost at replacement level, with an annual population growth rate of less than 1 per cent per year and it is still falling. The MMR is lower than that of countries at par with Sri Lanka as regards per capita income, and current maternal mortality is 30 deaths per 100,000 live births.

The success of Sri Lanka's health program, which in its early years targeted infant and maternal mortality and infectious and communicable diseases, is undeniable and is looked to by much of the world for the lessons it can teach. The World Bank has been working with the government of Sri Lanka toward this success, particularly in the reduction of communicable diseases. Having met several important challenges, Sri Lanka must now focus on solving the remaining major public health issues. Malnutrition among children and iron deficiency among pregnant and lactating women are still serious problems, and iodine deficiency may be more of a problem than is generally realized. Part of the population is still at risk of contracting malaria. Urgent steps must be taken to ensure that HIV prevalence in the population remains low. (World Bank, <http://www.worldbank.org>)

Meanwhile, of course, there have been changes—the burden of cardiovascular diseases, diabetes and other degenerative, non-communicable diseases has increased in the country, but the Sri Lankan government is planning to address these fresh challenges through the recently established Presidential Task Force on Health Reform.

India has to address many similar issues, and the progressive health indices that reflect improvement must be measured with a certain level of scepticism because they have a way of painting a rosy picture that hides the reality of the disease burden of the country. A third of the world's total burden of TB is in India, and of all the people who live with active TB, the largest number is in India. Malaria made a comeback in the late 1980s and settled at a fairly high rate of prevalence in the 1990s. Water-borne diseases like cholera, some forms of hepatitis and gastroenteritis remain serious health challenges. HIV/AIDS is a relatively new challenge, but very significant in its impact. Details of the current health burden that the country carries are discussed in Chapter 1 of this book. The problem is that as in Sri Lanka, globalization has brought with it an additional burden of diabetes, cardiovascular diseases, obesity and cancer. Complications related to blood pressure, cholesterol, and the intake of alcohol and tobacco have become a supplementary burden for countries like India.

While the inequality of nations and people is almost a philosophical truth which most world communities have generally accepted and live with, it is important that some of the basic reasons for India's lower position in the HDR, 2003 are identified and understood. One significant reason is the low health budget in India as compared to the world average. Health outcomes and the success of programmes in terms of real impact on peoples' health are strongly associated with the amount that is spent per capita on public health. This amount, as has been discussed in earlier chapters, is dismally low in India. Another important reason for India remaining on a lower rung in the global analysis of nations is poverty. While experts would like to have the world believe that the relationship between poverty and health is complex and multi-directional, it is actually very simple. The NHDR, 2001, which also lays emphasis on the complexity of this relationship, states how poor health can translate into impaired productivity of the human resource and also low earnings. Economists explain how poverty has declined but the health status of Indians has, on an average, not kept pace, and in fact, has remained quite low. This is a catch-22 situation—any future reduction in poverty is possible only if health status of the people is enhanced. Another prime reason for India remaining short of global standards is the fact that some large, but insulated, institutions and private health-care workers take pride in offering what they like to call 'world-class health care at nominal costs'. This recent phenomenon, a little over a decade old, has created a false sense of India having a finger in the global health-care pie. The point is, however, that this model is not on offer for the general well-being of ordinary Indian citizens simply because it is inaccessible to most. And, however many foreign patients may come to India for surgeries and specific treatments, India's position on the map is not going to change unless the country's health indices improve.

A large population size is also a significant contributor towards pushing the country down on any global monitoring scale. According to the Planning Commission, the coming two decades will witness an addition of at least 300 million people to the existing population (Planning Commission, 2002). Although fertility rates have declined in the country, so has infant mortality, and life expectancy has gone up remarkably. By 2020, India will have more than 1.3 billion people. The same period will see a doubling in the number of people over 60 years of age, a large number of illiterates, and people with special health needs. Although food production has grown phenomenally and will continue to grow, the problem we face today will remain: a lack of purchasing power among the people due to lack of employment opportunities. According to the *NHDR, 2001*, in the 1990s alone India's population has increased by 181 million—the equivalent of adding Australia's population each year to its own.

The current mismanagement and disorganization of existing human resources (Chapters 4 and 5) are other critical factors that hinder progress, keeping the country from achieving global equity and good standards of health care. It is also about setting realistic and achievable goals. The NHP of 2002 clearly shows how the earlier NHP (1983) hoped to bring in a golden period of 'health for all', only to be faced with harsh ground realities like the shortage of financial resources and administrative capacity of the public health system, necessary to achieve health for all. 'Against this backdrop, it is felt it would be appropriate to pitch NHP 2002 at a level consistent with our realistic expectations about financial resources, and about the likely increase in public health capacity' (*NHP, 2002*). For India, the constant gap between targets and achievements has been a huge internal problem that has affected the country's global standing. For every step that India has taken forward, it has not been easy to overcome the deeply entrenched inequality in human development that exists between developed and developing nations.

While much of the responsibility for such inequity can be squarely placed on the governments that have ruled the country over the last five decades and more, and on the equally responsible private sector that has steered clear of social responsibility over the years, focusing only on its immediate profits, there are other, external factors that cannot be ignored. It is also best understood that a global positioning has to be seen in the context of a country's peculiar condition and it need not be India's own failures alone that have pushed it into the position it is in today as far as public health delivery is concerned. The Director General of WHO, Dr Lee Jong-wook, says that the priorities of countries vary based on epidemiological patterns, and also on political choices, which is why WHO faces the constant challenge of making selective use of its limited resources. In a world that is marked by unacceptable health inequalities, WHO emphasizes those programmes that benefit the poorest and most vulnerable communities. Former Director General of WHO, Dr Gro Harlem Brundtland, has said in her message:

In poor countries today there are 170 million underweight

children, over three million of whom will die this year as a result. There are more than one billion adults worldwide who are overweight and at least 300 million who are clinically obese. Among these, about half a million people in North America and Western Europe combined will have died this year from obesity-related diseases. Could the contrast between the haves and the have-nots ever be more starkly illustrated? (*The World Health Report*, 2002)

Along with WHO, various international bodies have been trying to address this inequality, since there are multiple, and often very complex, reasons for the diverse standards in different countries. In September 2000, 147 nations met at a Millennium Summit to adopt what they called the Millennium Declaration, which sought to implement, in a time-bound fashion, the Millennium Development Goals—'an ambitious agenda for reducing poverty and improving lives' (UNDP, 2003). Keeping 1990 as the benchmark year, there are eight goals with eighteen quantifiable targets, with the deadlines for most being 2015 (For further information see Box: What the World Wants to Achieve, pp. 143–44). India too has its own plans to achieve specific targets through its Tenth Five Year Plan drawn up by the Planning Commission—these are relatively short-term goals to be achieved over the next five to ten years. Some of the health-specific targets are: to reduce the ratio of poverty by 5 per cent by 2007 and by 15 per cent by 2012; to bring down the decadal rate of population growth between 2001 and 2011 to 16.2 per cent; to reduce IMR to 45 per 1000 live births by 2007 and to 28 by 2012; and, to reduce the MMR to 2 per 1000 live births by 2007 and to 1 by 2012. There are also specific targets for HIV/AIDS: 80 per cent coverage of high-risk groups through targeted interventions; 90 per cent coverage of schools and colleges through education programmes; 80 per cent awareness among the general population in rural areas; reducing transmission through blood to less than 1 per cent; establishing at least one voluntary testing and counselling centre in every district; scaling up activities for the prevention of mother-to-child transmission activities up to the district level; achieving zero-level increase of HIV/AIDS prevalence by 2007. Specific targets to combat malaria include covering an Annual Blood Examination Rate (ABER) of over 10 per cent; working towards an Annual Parasite Incidence (API) of 1.3 or less; and reducing by a quarter the morbidity and mortality due to malaria by 2007 and halving the same by 2010 (*NHP, 2002*). According to the *HDR, 2003*, fifty-nine countries of the world may not be able to reach the goals set by the Millennium Summit by 2015. In fact, there are thirty-one countries where progress towards these goals has ceased or even shown a reversal. In India, overall progress has apparently been excellent, especially with goal 1, which is to eradicate extreme poverty and hunger, with the target being to halve the proportion of people suffering from hunger at present. Within India, though, this so-called progress must be approached with caution because, according to the *HDR*, 'some areas and groups are not benefiting enough, while wealthy segments of the population continue to surge ahead'. In goal 4, which is to reduce child mortality, the target was to reduce under-5 mortality and IMR by two-thirds. In the case of the former, India is lagging behind; Sri Lanka, on the other hand, is on track with both goals 1 and 4.

It is well known that the disparity is not just between the Indian and the global scene, it is also within the country, between states. State-wise inequity is important to note because the better-performing states could help bring India closer to global standards. It is an acknowledged fact that health attainments at the national level actually mask very significant inter- and intra-state differences (*NHDR, 2001*). The state of Kerala, often quoted as an example of world-class health attainments, is at one end of this spectrum of success. Using the democratic form of government to maximum advantage, and with the total absence of coercive practices, Kerala has achieved very high health indices, especially in the areas of birth and death rates, IMR and literacy. The IMR declined to 42 in 1991 and under-5 mortality was 80 per 1000. The proportion of births attended by health professionals was 88 per cent and 96 per cent in rural and urban parts of Kerala, while the same figure was 11 and 44 in Uttar Pradesh. But experts believe that these attainments will be hard to replicate in other states because of the kind of social reform and visionary movements that are peculiar to Kerala. The Christian missions, existence of a matriarchal society, rising age of marriage, high literacy levels, massive investment in health and eduction, and the rural–urban continuum in habitation have all been important contributors to the improved health scene. Many of Kerala's health indicators are comparable to those in middle-income countries, whereas in the states of Uttar Pradesh, Madhya Pradesh and Orissa health indices are almost at the level of sub-Saharan Africa. Yet, Kerala's new challenge is to be able to face up to the highest incidence of morbidity for acute and chronic ailments—a factor that always contrasts with mortality. In fact, according to a study by the World Bank, these differences between states will have to be closely considered and studied if they are to be of any use to the overall health-care system in the country (Peters et al., 2002). For instance, states like Kerala and Tamil Nadu will need to focus on:

introducing and expanding public health services for cardiovascular disease, mental health and injuries as these are now the prominent conditions facing their populations. Other states are earlier in the transition but should also consider selective interventions in these areas. For example, Orissa and West Bengal have very high rates of tobacco use, particularly among their poor. (Peters et. al., 2002)

In the larger scheme of the things, lack of basic health services and safe drinking water in the less-privileged countries remain a problem, according to the *HDR, 2003*. The incidence of HIV/AIDS is growing. In fact the United Nations Secretary-General, Kofi Annan, has brought to the attention of the world's top leaders, the Group of Eight, the need to work towards providing 'greater financial resources and trade opportunities for the developing world'. While world leaders agree that the Millennium Development Goals encapsulate the world's best chances of making things better, historical evidence shows otherwise: lofty, global directives and declarations have their strong limitations in being able to catalyse effective, local action. Nevertheless, with a lot of pride and enthusiasm, eighteen tangible and quantifiable targets have been drawn up to be able to sustain and monitor the Millennium Development Goals. According to the World Bank, India will become the fourth largest economy in the world by 2020. Whether or not it will also be able to scale similar heights in the health and well-being of its billion-plus population, is difficult to comment upon at present. The Planning Commission hopes, through *India Vision 2020*, that India will align some of its important health indices with those of upper- and middle-income (UMI) countries like Argentina, Chile, Hungary, Malaysia, Mexico and South Africa. It is a daunting task, even if one looks at a few of those indices: today, the percentage of people living below the poverty line is 26 per cent in India, and 13 per cent in the UMIs; female adult literacy rate is 44 per cent in India and 94 per cent in the UMIs; life expectancy at birth is 64 in India, 69 in the UMIs; infant mortality is 71 per 1000 live births in India and 22.5 in the UMIs; and child malnutrition as a percentage of children under 5 years of age, based on the weight-for-age, is 45 in India and 8 in the UMIs. And here is the Planning Commission's view on these challenges:

> We are confident that we can and will meet these challenges. We also feel that we have the knowledge and the capacity as a nation to achieve food for all, health for all, and jobs for all. What we do not know for sure however is, how long it will take us to accomplish them. We need, therefore, to affirm the will and determination to do it rapidly and achieve it now rather than sometime later. (Planning Commission, 2002)

Meanwhile, the world and India's people are waiting and watching, and while international comparisons always need to be drawn with caution since demographic realities are so different in each region, there are certainly a lot of lessons for India to learn.

WHAT THE WORLD WANTS TO ACHIEVE
The Millennium Development Goals
(Reproduced from <http://www.un.org/millenniumgoals/>)

Goal 1. Eradicate extreme poverty and hunger
Target for 2015: The number of people subsisting on less than a dollar a day, and suffering eternal hunger, will be halved.

Goal 2. Achieve universal primary education
Target for 2015: All young boys and girls will be completing primary school.

Goal 3. Promote gender equality and empower women
Targets for 2005 and 2015: Eliminate gender disparities in primary and secondary education preferably by 2005, and at all levels by 2015.

Goal 4. Reduce child mortality
Target for 2015: Reduce by two-thirds the mortality rate among children under 5.

Goal 5. Improve maternal health
Target for 2015: Reduce by three-quarters the ratio of women dying in childbirth.

Goal 6. Combat HIV/AIDS, malaria and other diseases
Target for 2015: Halt and begin to reverse the spread of HIV/AIDS and the incidence of malaria and other major diseases.

Goal 7. Ensure environmental sustainability
Targets: Integrate the principles of sustainable development into country policies and programmes and reverse the loss of environmental resources; by 2015, reduce by half the proportion of people without access to safe drinking water; by 2020 achieve significant improvement in the lives of at least 100 million slum dwellers.

Goal 8. Develop a global partnership for development
Targets: Develop further an open trading and financial system that includes a commitment to good governance, development and poverty reduction—nationally and internationally; address the least developed countries' special needs, and the special needs of landlocked and small island developing states; deal comprehensively with developing countries' debt problems; develop decent and productive work for youth; provide access to affordable essential drugs in developing countries in cooperation with pharmaceutical companies; and make available the benefits of new technologies—especially information and communications technologies—in cooperation with the private sector.

Town Mouse, Country Mouse

In an ongoing battle between hospital-centred technocentric
health care versus people-centred empowering health care,
we are trying to tilt the balance towards people by way of
research and demonstration.

—Dr Abhay Bang, Society for Education, Action and
Research in Community Health (SEARCH) in VHAI, 1998

There are cities, and then there are villages. Mostly, there
are villages. Hundreds of thousands of villages (638,365
according to the *Census of India, 2001*) spread across the
length and breadth of this enormous country, with a large
section of the population living, working and dying there.
Several deaths here are avoidable, but occur simply because
of lack of health-care amenities that ought to be available to
all people—villagers or city dwellers, mofussil town residents
or slum dwellers. But then, the village is just that to a lot of
people: a village. And life in the Indian village is lived on the
periphery of government attention, in a twilight zone where
a long list of amenities that are otherwise taken for granted
just do not exist. This is a fact that most thinking people are
well aware of, but feel rather helpless about. It is an issue
that comes up at conferences and heated, intellectual debates,

but few people lose any sleep over it. For, if that had happened, things would have been different for rural India. That it did happen to a handful has made a difference, and that tiny group of motivated people is trying to change the circumstances in which the rural folk of India live. Drs Abhay and Rani Bang are somewhere at the forefront of that motley group, and the total inadequacy of rural infrastructure made them set out in the late 1980s on a path less travelled—to the little-known, backward, east Maharashtra district of Gadchiroli. Here they found that health was one of the most seriously neglected areas of village life, and thus began their SEARCH for solutions.

It was a tough, long and arduous road for the aptly named SEARCH. The district, with a majority of tribals of the Madia Gond, faced all sorts of health challenges: a high incidence of RTIs and diseases among the women; alcoholism and reproductive health problems among the men; neonatal morbidity; and sickle cell anaemia (VHAI, 1998). It did not take the Bangs long to realize what they were up against— abysmally poor health care and very high child mortality; civil surgeons posted in the region who spent an average of five days each month in Gadchiroli; and a thirty-bed district hospital where no successful caesarean section for child delivery had ever been performed. Over the two eventful decades that have followed, SEARCH's work has found shape and substance. The approach is based on carrying out basic community-level research to identify the problems of the people, and then to go on and develop appropriate solutions. Interestingly, the beginnings of this organization were in collaboration with the government structure. The Bangs took over the running of two PHCs, but working with the public sector soon became difficult for reasons that are so well known as regards health services in rural areas.

Finally, the Bangs found themselves running the whole show. The irony is that the health department found this so embarrassing that SEARCH became more like an adversary, almost a threat to the cosy complacency in which many government departments function, or do not function. While SEARCH set out on its own, there was also the realization that the government was 'working not to meet the felt needs of the people, but to meet its own targets'.

This is the scenario in the majority of health-care institutions in the villages across rural India. Besides this lack of prioritization of the special needs of rural people, there is also the more troubling aspect of rural health care—empty hospitals devoid of equipment, doctors and paramedical staff. Debates in the top echelons centre around how India needs to achieve world standards in health care, but the reality is that while some Indians can access the best medical care from top-of-the-rung professionals in globally competitive hospital settings, there is the other India where even the most basic services—from vaccinations to protect children from common communicable diseases to a safe haven where a mother can deliver her baby and still go home alive and well—are not found for the love of money. According to the *NHDR, 2001*, the rural–urban divide is as evident as the gender divide. India's growing mountains of publicly held food stocks notwithstanding, food and nutritional security at the household level continue to be a dream for a substantial section of the population, especially those who live in the villages and urban slums, and in the peripheries of townships. The irony is that this other India is almost two-thirds of the population. It is also unfortunate because the government had taken great pains to put in place in the 1980s a huge network of PHCs and CHCs for rural areas (VHAI, 1997). Today, the network still exists, is even growing, but its ability to reach out to and enhance the health of the rural population has never needed to be questioned more than it is now. That urban areas are much better endowed with public health facilities than rural India is a known fact (Duggal, 2001).

The challenges that rural folk face in terms of health and well-being are not very different from the health problems of urban folk. It is a similarity that may surprise, even disturb, many city dwellers who have distanced themselves so painstakingly from villages and villagers. Diarrhoeal diseases, TB and morbidity from cold and cough are common causes of ill health. According to Shariff, 'incidence of TB is 32 per cent higher in the less developed villages whereas leprosy is 200 per cent higher' (Shariff, 1999). Diarrhoea is common among the scheduled tribes and low among rural women— the higher the income and adult literacy rate, the lower is the prevalence of diarrhoea. Hypertension is also a common condition. ARIs, viral hepatitis, cholera, malaria and conditions peculiar to childhood are also major health problems targeting rural people. With the overall circumstances in which this huge rural majority lives, the same health conditions which could have easily been cured in the cities can become life-threatening in the villages. In fact, the government itself admits to significant gaps in the health indices between urban and rural populations, so much so that it is disturbing to note the ease with which this admittance is made. Infant mortality is 75 per 1000 live births in rural areas as compared to 44 in urban areas (NHP, 2002); in rural areas 103.7 children under 5 years die for every 1000 who live, and this figure is 63.1 in urban areas.

According to the NHP, 2002: 'While there is a general shortage of medical personnel in the country, this shortfall is disproportionately impacted on the less-developed and rural areas.' The VHAI conducted a survey and found that less than 20 per cent of the rural population has access to allopathic medicines, pushing basic surgical services to a far-off goalpost. In fact, any kind of medical care that is technology-intensive is all the more limited. According to the *NHDR, 2001*, this lack of access to basic health care in the villages has been exacerbated by the fact that the health-care sector itself has been preoccupied with 'maintenance and strengthening of private health-care services, perhaps, on account of the inertia of colonial inheritance'. This has been at the 'expense of broadening and deepening the public health-care system targeted at controlling the incidence of disease, particularly communicable diseases, in rural areas'. Little wonder then that there are very significant rural–urban disparities in various mortality, morbidity and nutrition indicators. According to the *NFHS-2*, basic coverage of preventive health programmes by the state has been much lower in rural as compared to urban areas. Completed vaccinations, for instance, had covered 60.5 per cent of urban areas, as compared to only 36.6 per cent of rural areas. The BCG vaccine administration programme showed similar discrepancies in terms of its coverage: 86.5 per cent (urban) and 67.1 per cent (rural); with DPT-3 vaccine, it was 73.4 per cent (urban) and 49.8 per cent (rural). The frustrations of village folk are therefore totally justified and understandable.

SEARCH has been very successful in tackling many basic health issues, but their experience with ARIs in children has been exceptional. Their decade-old publication in *Lancet*, the prestigious medical science journal from the United Kingdom, became a blueprint for global ARI control. Within two years of their beginning work in 1989–90, two-thirds of the deaths from pneumonia in children ceased, infant mortality in general went down by 33 per cent, and child mortality by 30 per cent. Their method was simple case management with the help of trained village *dais* and workers who diagnosed and treated pneumonia in children as it occurred. In fact, they even experimented with treating newborn babies, otherwise considered a risky business. Their resounding success prompted private doctors practising in the area to call in traditional health workers to cure patients of pneumonia.

If individual organizations can achieve success, why cannot the government do the same? Considering the enormous network that has been put in place to deliver good health across the length and breadth of the country, what has gone wrong? The reasons are so clear that they do not really require repeating: inadequate availability of resources; lack of basic equipment; lack of medicines and essential manpower in the public health system of rural areas; lack of availability of affordable care; and, most importantly, the inability of the central government and the states to prioritize the health-care needs of the village people. Just as the Bangs found first-hand, it also has a lot to do with individual motivation among doctors who are posted to the 'rural outback'; for most, this is something to wriggle out of by any means. Earlier analyses have shown just how much discrepancy there is between the number of specialist posts that are required in these areas, the actual number sanctioned and, finally, the number actually in position. Less than a decade ago, the number of surgeons required across India's CHCs was 2401, 1353 posts were sanctioned and, the actual number of surgeons in position was 710. The number of paediatricians required were the same as those of surgeons, of which 845 were sanctioned and just 498 were in position (VHAI, 1997). It would be intriguing to see the results of a survey of all doctors to find out the frequency and duration of rural postings over their entire career span of thirty to thirty-five years! But for many villagers, the doctor comes later—just reaching the PHC/CHC for them is a journey fraught with many problems. Each sub-primary health centre is at least 2 kilometres away for every villager, and a PHC about 5 kilometres away. But whether the centre has a doctor on its staff or not is really an existential question for many.

Another serious issue that confronts people in the villages is the cost of curative health care, and their inability to tackle the mushrooming of private health care and the prohibitive costs it brings in its wake. The skewed movement of people towards the more expensive option of curing disease has been almost simultaneous in the villages and the cities. For instance, the percentage of people using public health-care facilities for in-patient care was 45.3 per cent in the villages and 43.1 per cent in urban areas; similarly, out-patient care was 19 per cent for rural areas and 20 per cent for urban areas (*NSS*, 1995–96). Just as people run to private practitioners in the city, disillusioned by the large, public city-hospital, so is the case in many villages. This trend has proved very costly, and has come about for two reasons: the first is the inadequacy of preventive health programmes, and the second is the aggressive marketing of curative health care by the private sector. 'On an average, rural households spend 4 per cent of their total income on the treatment of common ailments, but the poor spend about 9 per cent of their total income. This is despite the delivery of free health care services by the government' (Shariff, 1999). The *India: Human Development Report* (1999) by the NCAER, New Delhi, was produced at the end of a multipurpose survey of 33,000 households in rural India, spread over 1765 villages and 195 districts in sixteen Indian states (January–May 1994). The economic burden of treating disease is enormous in rural India, and the really poor can spend up to 20 per cent of their total annual income in search of good health alone. As Shariff explains in his report, the rich may spend more in absolute terms on health care, but it is an 'insignificant proportion in relation to their household income'. People who earn more than Rs 86,000 a year spend only 0.6 per cent of this income on health care; but in families where annual earnings are less than Rs 20,000, the expenditure on health is 8.3 per cent of their income. 'This clearly underscores the importance and need for public health services for the poorer sections of the population' (Shariff, 1999). The government might quickly point towards all the services that are in place—so what if they are ghost buildings with no doctors, no medicine supplies, and no equipment. The point is, it has to be a vibrant, alive, functioning network, not just figures on a graph in an official report.

So, what can be done? Spruce up the PHC/CHC network and fill the buildings with real people, that is, qualified doctors? Bring in equipment that works, and keep it working? Stock the empty, cobwebbed cupboards with basic medical amenities and drugs? Motivate health workers enough to walk the many extra miles, work without electricity or potable water, and stay in touch with each villager? The need is for larger systemic change—something that has always proved very challenging, expensive and difficult to achieve. But smaller, local solutions that can work at micro-societal levels have always helped make things better in both rural and urban areas. Whatever the methodology of intervention, if fuelled by motivation to fulfil the needs of a community, these solutions can work wonders. They can be simple interventions, such as the one tried by the Sri Chithra Thirunal Institute for Medical Sciences and Technology in Thiruvananthapuram, Kerala, where Dr Thankappan and others have attempted to involve the panchayati raj institutions in handing out health care to villagers. This is a workable idea simply because a panchayat knows the trials and tribulations of a village much better than anybody else, is able to address the needs of the village in a much more focussed way, and can do so with much greater efficiency. Now, the *NHP, 2002* hopes to replicate similar examples across the country, not just in rural areas but also in cities.

Some states have adopted a policy of devolving programmes and funds in the health sector through different levels of the panchayati raj institutions. Generally, the experience has been an encouraging one. The adoption of such an organizational structure has enabled need-based allocation of resources and closer supervision through elected representatives. The Policy examines the need for a wider adoption of this mode of delivery of health services, in rural as well as urban areas, in other parts of the country. (*NHP, 2002*)

There are many other examples of how people are trying to change the health-care scene in rural India. In 1993, the Association of Rural Surgeons of India (ARSI) was formed as a network to provide 'viable models of rural health care that is accessible and affordable to a common person'. There is also the Small Scale Rural Surgical Clinics (SSRSC) in West Bengal (*NHDR, 2001*). The situation today is such that more than half the operations (60 per cent) are being conducted by these small clinics, with the state-run, sub-divisional hospital absorbing the remaining 40 per cent. Medical care is provided at a fraction of the normal cost by a lone qualified and experienced doctor, supported by a locally trained team of paramedics, and often without the help of a trained anaesthetist. Offering similar, affordable care is the Rural

Medicare Society in the suburbs of Delhi, providing both preventive and curative medical care.

For Dr H.R. Sudarshan, winner of the 1994 Right Livelihood Award, this search for solutions has been a long one but with light at the end of the tunnel. Through the experiences of the Vivekananda Girijana Kalyana Kendra (VGKK) that he set up in 1981 in the Biligiri Rangana hills of Mysore in Karnataka, he has seen that success is elusive unless an integrated community development programme approach is followed. Dr Sudarshan, Project Director of VGKK, has followed this approach to improve the lives of the Soliga tribe in the region. When he began his work in this deprived region, infant mortality was around 150 per 1000 live births, and roughly 20 per cent of the children in the area were severely malnourished (VHAI, 1991). Slowly over the next decade, the IMR came down to 75 per 1000 live births and severe malnourishment came down to 4 per cent. It has been a remarkable two decades now, and to many observers and experts, what the VGKK has achieved is 'far beyond any that government efforts could ever have'. Leprosy is down from 17 per 1000 people to less that 0.3. Affordable cataract operations are being done routinely, bringing down the incidence of premature blindness. Dr Sudarshan now works closely with the government of Karnataka on health reform in the state.

The most important aspect of rural health care is that it has to be people-friendly and attuned to the cultural and social sensitivities of the target population who live simply without the many complexities of city life. The same principle was followed when the Bangs built Shodha Gram, a hospital for tribals which is constructed and managed in a way that is familiar to the tribals so that they don't find themselves in a strange environment. When SEARCH began its work, the area it covered was fifty-eight villages and 50,000 people. Health care is brought to these people through trained community health workers called arogyadoots (messenger of health). The Bangs' effort has been unique because they have managed to string in an active research component into their programme. Here too they redefined the choice and dimensions of their research based on what the people thought needed researching.

SEARCH tried various options. Working in partnership with the government was among the first methods, as already mentioned. But when the government decided to brand SEARCH as a meddler rather than a partner in strength, the Bangs realized that unless the locals of Gadchiroli could be roped in, there would be no hope for success. For, if the people were involved, they would see first-hand the extent of improvement and would realize that it was not some transient phenomenon that could die out any day. Unfortunately, more often than not the government reacts negatively to such local partnerships with NGOs. But it is perhaps only partnerships, non-government and government, that can really take health care to the villages. The government itself admits that reaching private health care to the rural areas is a Herculean, if not impossible, task (NHP, 2002). And getting private health care to the villages may not be the solution either as it is just too expensive. The NHP of 2002 has mooted the idea that this problem can be solved only if a paramedical set-up is created in full force, with good nurses and support medical staff trained to function as full-fledged public health experts and even doctors, or if a SEARCH or a VGKK is cloned in every rural district. One cannot but hope for a couple like the Bangs for every city and town. After all, life in the urban slum, however far removed it may be from the village, is devoid of good and efficient health care as well. In fact, the situation of people in urban slums or satellite towns of mega cities is in some ways worse because they suffer the additional burden of city environments—pollution and road accidents, in particular—without any special care to protect them from these dangers to health and safety. These twilight-zone urban areas too need innovative methods to reach health care to them, and a SEARCH or a VGKK would make a world of difference to them. The most powerful aspect of programmes such as these is the simplicity of their approach, driven as they are by genuine concern, respect for local problems, and a real desire to solve them.

Making it Work

The ultimate responsibility for the overall performance of
a country's health system lies with [the] government, which
in turn should involve all sectors of society in its
stewardship. The careful and responsible management of
the well-being of the population is the very essence of good
government. For every country it means establishing the
best and fairest health system possible with available
resources. The health of the people is always a national
priority: government responsibility for it is continuous and
permanent. Ministries of health must therefore take on a
large part of the stewardship of health systems.

—*The World Health Report*, 2000

In the central Indian city of Indore stands a large government-
owned hospital, a half-century-old building where the sick
throng in multitudes to seek relief from disease. However,
the Maharaja Yashwantrao Hospital (MYH) had received,
till recently, more recognition as a haven for rodents! But the
point is that it was really a large and popular hospital, the
rats notwithstanding. It has seven storeys and 800 beds, and
for all its reputation, MYH had anywhere between 10,000–
15,000 patients walking the corridors, queuing up in the out-

patients department and being admitted in the many wards. Then, something happened to change the way things were at MYH, so radically and so completely that it was almost as though the old hospital had been razed to the ground and a new one built in its place. The clean-up operation of this hospital was not just a logistical challenge, but also the beginning of a health-reform movement that brought welcome change not just in the city of Indore, but across the state of Madhya Pradesh. And somewhere, every person involved in this revolution knew that the beginning of change was not the real issue, but sustaining and maintaining that change was the biggest and the toughest challenge. In this chapter, an attempt is made to (a) bring together a few such experiences from across India by detailing their genesis and growth, and (b) to discuss how these experiences can be used to overcome the hurdles towards achieving better health and health care in India.

The Non-governmental Force for Change

According to VHAI, voluntary health care in India carries with it a certain historical baggage: the complete neglect of traditional systems of health care during the colonial era (VHAI, 1997). Most health activities were carried out by Christian missionaries, with the exception being the teachings and practices of Mahatma Gandhi who always laid great emphasis on traditional Indian systems of healing, especially naturopathy and yoga. Till the mid-1960s, according to VHAI, voluntary health care was restricted to hospital-based solutions provided by family trusts and charities or religious institutions. This was also the time when the concept of curative care was beginning to be seriously debated, and China was starting to show the way in terms of effective decentralized care through active involvement of the local community. Today, the entire voluntary health-care sector functions through community health programmes run by NGOs, by the government, by NGOs working for the government, and through social groups and individual activists who sponsor and directly involve themselves in community-based health work.

Indore's MYH owes its new lease of life to an interesting mix of all these approaches practised by the Rogi Kalyan Samiti (RKS), an NGO, pushing for better health across Madhya Pradesh. The beginnings of the RKS were tough and, as is always the case with institutions that try and revolutionize old and well-established systems, enormously challenging. But there was somebody who was catalysing this change: a young and dynamic officer from the Indian Administrative Service (IAS). His motivation helped strengthen a citizen's cadre that rose to the occasion and took charge. The state government was very supportive and provided active assistance wherever it could; wherever it couldn't, it stepped back and allowed RKS to function. All these combined to create a health-care revolution at MYH—a change for the better that stands as one of the best examples of how an NGO can become a prime force especially if it can work in partnership with the government. It all started in 1994, when S.R. Mohanty came to Indore as Collector. In charge of various government departments as their chief administrator, Mohanty led a busy life. That is when the plague epidemic broke out in Surat, and since Indore is less than 200 kilometres away from Surat, he decided to undertake a huge clean-up drive in his city. It didn't take much imagination to figure out where Mohanty would need to start—it had to be MYH, the derelict, dirty, giant building that was supposed to be the source of health care for Indore's people. Mohanty still cringes when he looks back. 'There were rats everywhere. The hospital had thousands of rodents, hundreds of tonnes of garbage, junk lying everywhere and deplorable service. It was no surprise that the average citizen was mortally afraid of entering a public hospital like the MYH' (personal conversation with S.R. Mohanty). Mohanty has some pictures in his collection that would make anybody shudder, pictures of a patient lying in bed with an intravenous drip and a rat poised on the bedstead, almost watching over the tubes and monitors!

Mohanty was overwhelmed. He knew he had to set things right, and this knowledge stemmed from an incident in his early childhood. His father had rushed a mortally wounded driver who worked for them to a hospital in their home-state, Orissa. Mohanty, then ten years old, had accompanied his father and was appalled at the filth cluttering the hospital. He wondered how anybody could fight for life in a place that looked like a garbage dump. The driver died eventually due to a lack of quick and proper medical attention, and now, looking back, Mohanty believes that the incident was a significant source of motivation for the kind of health-care reform he has managed to undertake in Indore. He knew that setting MYH right would be a challenge for an IAS officer, something almost impossible to achieve unless he got the people of the city involved in it. About 120 leading citizens got together to create a general body and decided, with Mohanty's guidance, to go ahead and complete the project of cleaning up MYH without any financial assistance from the government. As it turned out, money was the least of their problems because from the initial stages of the project, funds started pouring in as donations from the people of Indore. But before any activity could begin, patients were evacuated to eight hospitals in other parts of the city (Mohanty, 2001).

It took the help of 500 paid and voluntary workers to fill up 150 trucks of garbage for disposal. But compared to the rats, clearing the junk was easy. The anti-rodent drive had to be conducted in a much more logical and scientific manner, and for all his strengths, Mohanty found he was no Pied Piper. Workers spent days and weeks identifying burrows, filling them with poisonous bait, spraying circles of poison around the periphery of the building, sealing all sewers and, finally, letting poisonous gas into the sealed hospital building. The rat graveyard that the workers found soon after was a terribly unpleasant sight, but it made Mohanty and his team happy to see their local technology actually working. After this, thousands of dead rodents were consigned to an incinerator and the hospital was cleaned up with active assistance from the fire department. The MYH was reborn. Space in the sprawling building was reallocated rationally, so that operation theatres doubling up as office space were restored to what they were meant to be. An emergency ward of 100 beds was created without any additional construction, doctors' consultation rooms that had come up in private wards were cleared out, and at least forty rooms were reclaimed during the clean-up and allocated to specialists to run their clinics. Administrative reform was also brought in, and according to Mohanty, this is always a serious weak link in the running of many large health-care institutions in India. Routine hospital management can be a great challenge and the RKS worked hard to put systems in place at the MYH so as to allow for the smooth running of the hospital.

But very soon Mohanty realized that all the hard work would be useless if it could not be sustained over time, with or without him. A vital factor that would help achieve sustenance, Mohanty knew instinctively, was to levy a user charge or registration fee. It was this factor, along with the need to administer the hospital with efficiency, that led to the formation of the RKS, which literally means the patient welfare committee. In Mohanty's mind, the RKS was to have a simple and straight mandate—a people's body to monitor the hospital's day-to-day running. A management system that was participatory in its approach was introduced, with the RKS overseeing all activities. According to Mohanty, the MYH became the first government hospital in the state of Madhya Pradesh to levy two kinds of charges, one very nominal fee for the general patient and another slightly higher slab for private-ward patients. As it is across India, even the amount for private-ward patients is much less than what private hospitals charge. Care for people below the poverty line is free. Of course, to avail of free care, a patient needs to go through a formal procedure of self-certification so as to ensure that he or she really does not have the means to pay for treatment. But this too must be followed through. The RKS is based on mutual human trust and faith and as Mohanty says: 'In studies done over the years we have found to our pleasant surprise that the number of infringements of this faith have been insignificant—well below one per cent.' A far cry from what is seen in large, corporate hospitals in the mega cities, where non-eligible patients utilize the free health-care facilities with the help of fake documents. It is also not surprising that the fees have not deterred patients who throng the MYH; if anything, the new-look hospital now attracts more patients, both in in-patient and out-patient departments.

Mohanty believes that the deplorable condition that the MYH was in before the clean-up operation was due to a combination of factors, an important one being the amount of funding it received each year, a paltry Rs 1.8 lakh as contingency allocation grant. While that remains the same, what has changed is that the RKS pitches in with a substantial

Rs 52 lakh each year. But there is also the larger malaise, a lack of strong and clear governance of the public health infrastructure. As Mohanty himself says:

> There was a time when the Additional Collector of Indore was admitted in the Intensive Cardiac Care Unit of MYH and had rodents running all over him; there was a time when a pig picked up a newborn baby in Lady Butler Hospital and chewed it to death even before the family could be informed of the birth. (Mohanty, 2001)

Now things are different. Across Madhya Pradesh, more than 600 hospitals have established RKS units; more than 6000 citizens are now part of these societies, managing large government hospitals. Today the RKS is part of state policy and has become a workable solution to one of India's biggest health challenges: running a large, state hospital efficiently and providing basic health-care facilities to all.

Non-governmental efforts in trying to bring in change are also very often found to be effective when health care has been juxtaposed with larger community-based reform, such as empowering women through microcredit self-help groups, or encouraging women to attend night school, or spreading literacy, general awareness and knowledge. For the multi-faceted Self-Employed Women's Association (SEWA), known among the fashion-conscious for the Lucknow chikankari work they produce and sell as ready-to-wear clothing and fabric, providing health care is very straight forward: volunteers make door-to-door visits and offer simple preventive health care and immunization. Providing rational drugs at low prices, childcare services for working women, and ensuring constant interaction with home-based women have been SEWA's unique selling points, and they seem to have worked. The Indian woman, even in urban areas, is bashful and reluctant, and this fact becomes one of the biggest challenges to the country's health system. According to SEWA:

> SEWA has helped its members obtain health care which is run by women themselves. Our approach emphasizes health education as well as curative care. It also involves coordination and collaboration with government health services for immunization, micronutrient supplementation, family planning, tuberculosis control and referral care at public hospitals, dispensaries and primary health centres. <http://www. sewa.org>

SEWA has designed its health programme in such a way that health is intimately linked to the ability to make a living and to the economics of life.

It has been found that making women self-reliant in their earning capacity can also strengthen their ability to take charge of their lives and take care of their health and that of their families. It is a highly decentralized programme, run largely by the women of the community who have started functioning as midwives, health workers for immunizations, promoters of contraceptive methods and sources of information and awareness about the importance of health and nutrition. But it is important to highlight some factors that have made these successes what they are. At SEWA, health care—preventive health services, immunization, and rational drug supply at low prices—and childcare is provided to its members through two health cooperatives, the Mahila Sewa Lok Swasthya Cooperative (MSLSC) and the Krishna Dayan Cooperative (KDC) (Panchamukhi and Nayak, 2001). Health insurance coverage is extended to those members who make contributions. Members who link their fixed deposit savings with the insurance scheme also get coverage for maternity benefit. The SEWA bank runs the Integrated Social Security Insurance Scheme (ISSIS) with the help of the Life Insurance Corporation (LIC) of India and United India Insurance (UII) (Rs 70–80 is paid as premium per year). Studies have shown that out-of-pocket expenses of insured households were at least 30 per cent less for chronic and acute diseases and less by 60 per cent for hospitalization. 'We found the only really effective way to reach out would be to actually go door to door, so that is what we do now,' says Usha Parekh of SEWA. SEWA has scored in being able to organize traditional *dais* into cohesive groups, and in ensuring not only that the midwife is available for those who need her, but also that she gets her due for the service she has rendered to society over the ages. *Dais* are, in a sense, wonderful barefoot doctors.

At the Barefoot College in Tilonia, Rajasthan, Dr Bunker Roy, a well-known social worker, has been trying to bring about change through the famous barefoot revolution and has made doctors out of ordinary, village folk. Historically, it was in the 1960s that the barefoot doctors of China started to make an impact in alleviating the health scenario in rural China <http://www.infochangeindia.org>. At Tilonia too, the basic spirit remains the same, which is to empower ordinary folk with the essential skills, intellectual power and technical know-how to be able to manage their lives without professional help from the cities, which is anyway hard to get.

Also kicking off their shoes was a doctor-couple, Drs Nandakumar and Shylaja Menon, originally from India but working in state-of-the-art hospitals in New York, who arrived at the Gudalur Adivasi Hospital in Gudalur in the Nilgiris in Tamil Nadu more than a decade ago <http://www.infochangeindia.org>. Working among the adivasis in the region, these two committed doctors found satisfaction in the fact that whatever they were doing showed positive results—diarrhoeal deaths hardly occur anymore, infant and maternal mortality figures are better than the national average, and health is no longer a distant dream for many of these hill people.

For over a century at least, sex work has flourished in Sonagachi, Kolkata, where today at least 15,000 sex workers live and work. Back in the early 1990s, a collaboration between the All India Institute of Hygiene and Public Health in Kolkata, WHO, and the National AIDS Control Organization resulted in an operational research programme that was initially meant to study the prevalence of STDs and HIV infection among sex workers. More than 80 per cent of the sex workers were suffering from some sexually transmitted infection or the other and hardly any client used a condom. The study led to an intervention programme designed to reduce infection in the community. The programme involved sex workers at the core of its functioning and did not work through preaching from the outside. Peer educators of the Sonagachi Project are sex workers themselves, who make house visits and talk about the need to use condoms and the threat of STDs. Sonagachi's success has also been projected as a role model for others to follow, especially because it has also empowered the women of the community in more ways than one. There is an organized set-up with women members from other parts of the state of West Bengal. They now have a global presence, and as part of worldwide networks they participate in international conferences, work through an active cooperative so that they are economically protected, speak up for the rights of sex workers, and ensure their recognition as a labour force in India (Ranjita Biswas, <http://www.sdnp.undp.org>, September 1999). According to one of the documentations of the Sonagachi Project:

Right from the beginning we adopted a very flexible approach so that we could adapt the programme to the changing circumstances and needs articulated by the community we worked with. In this way we could remodel it when necessary, as our perceptions were enriched by our growing experience of working with the sex workers' community. The STD/HIV Intervention Programme (SHIP) popularly known as the Sonagachi Project has been able to control STD and HIV transmission among sex workers and their sexual partners since its inception in 1992. Data from the latest evaluative survey done in 1999 are as follows: positivity for venereal disease has changed from 25.4 in 1992 to 11.5. Genital ulcer prevalence has reduced from 6.22 in 1992 to 0.99. HIV prevalence has remained stable within 5 per cent during 1995 to 1998, which is remarkably low for this community. Condom use has increased from 2.7 in 1992 to 80.5 per cent in 1998. (Jana et al., 1999)

The strength of the Sonagachi Project was that the people who conducted the intervention were able to respond to the target community's real needs. And in India, this can be an enormous challenge considering the level of illiteracy and lack of awareness among various communities as regards their own health and well-being.

While many groups are working across the country to break these barriers, some have been very successful. The People's Health Movement (PHM) in Kerala, run by the well-known Kerala Sastra Sahitya Parishad (KSSP), organizes health classes for villagers. These classes focus on diseases that are rampant in specific areas of the state, and on nutrition and basics like first-aid. Over the years, the KSSP has realized that though Kerala has set examples for the country on meeting developmental goals, poverty and diseases related to it are still rampant. This led the organization to carry out what is to date considered to be a landmark survey of 10,000 rural homes. *Health and Development in Rural Kerala* (Kannan et. al, 1991) surveyed not just the state of health in rural homes but also the institution of urban health care in the form of hospitals and the health-care delivery system. They found that although Kerala had worked hard on achieving very low birth and death rates, a high female sex ratio and low infant mortality, there was still a high rate of morbidity from various diseases. This was because despite the achievements in literacy and awareness, economic backwardness continued to dog the state.

The KSSP was formed in 1959 to bring science and society together in the literate and educated state of Kerala, and it took many years to find its way into the health sector. It was in 1977 (VHAI, 1999) that the KSSP's work in the health sector began and the PHM gathered momentum soon after. As is common in Kerala, there was a significant involvement of traditional health systems in this movement, such as the ayurveda school, along with allopathic specialists. The KSSP has strongly criticized the NHP and also the general direction that the government's health sector has taken as far as its development is concerned. Trying to bring back the old definition of public health, the KSSP has been arguing persistently that while India's current health structure is built on the 'doctor, drugs and hospitals' approach, there should be a focus on nutrition, safe drinking water, education and employment. This falls in line with their philosophy (which they have constantly articulated) that the medical profession and big hospitals are not the core of the health sector; in fact, it is socio-economic reform. This would of course hardly be music to the ears of many of the country's health professionals. The uniqueness of the KSSP lies in the fact that it is really a mass, state-wide movement that has managed to diversify its mandate as an organization working to make life better in more ways than one.

In fact, as has been the KSSP's experience, a large number of health NGOs across India have found what could be the 'best practice': just empower the people with knowledge and then step back. The Urmul Trust in Rajasthan has tried to put forth a simple, step-wise method of tackling malaria epidemics: recognize the fever and act without delay. The Mahila Sarvangeen Utkarsh Mandal (MASUM) in Pune run by Manisha Gupte has a similar philosophy: understand your health and then do something about it. MASUM trains women to become health workers, and also pushes aggressively for self-examination as a major factor that can help women control their health status.

Cancer support groups throughout the country are working along similar lines to empower people with knowledge and then provide them with whatever support they need to tackle this difficult disease. The Mumbai-based Cancer Patients Aid Association (CPAA) has made a difference to the lives of at least 40,000 cancer patients <http://www.infochangeindia.org>. A large part of their work involves arranging for finances for cancer treatment, counselling patients and families, helping patients in need of surgery to get blood or prostheses with ease, and providing assistance for travel and stay in Mumbai during the course of treatment. Considering the magnitude of India's health problems, every effort counts.

At the Shankara Netralaya in Chennai, a state-of-the-art eye hospital, 40 per cent of the patients are treated free of cost. What fuels the institution is a question many ask. Certainly not money, and at a time when India is witnessing a mushrooming of corporate-style hospitals that very few can really afford, this comes as a surprise. Named after the Shankaracharya of Kanchi and established in 1978, the hospital today is an ISO 9002 certified institution and offers the same quality of service to those who can afford it and those who cannot.

The Impact of Effective Government Programmes

As WHO puts forth in completely unambiguous terms (*The World Health Report*, 2000), the real responsibilities for looking after the health needs of a nation's people and of running a health-care programme effectively lie with the government. But in India, the government has not been able to stay abreast of the country's health needs, primarily because of large-scale mismanagement of the enormous public health-care infrastructure, an indifferent attitude to the health-care needs of the people, and the low priority accorded to health care by political parties. And yet, there are many instances where the government has managed to make significant impact on improving health systems, either by providing solid, external support to non-governmental programmes and organizations, or by carrying out specific government programmes with targeted goals.

The RKS experiment in Indore, for instance, received tremendous support from the government of Madhya Pradesh and the chief minister, and it is well known that a large part of its success was a result of this support. The government has also had spectacular success with individual programmes in the last few decades. The intensive Pulse Polio Programme was launched by the government in 1995 to cover every child under the age of 5 years with the Oral Polio Vaccine on National Immunization Days and Sub-national Immunization Days. Over the last few years, the government has stepped up these efforts and according to the MHFW *Annual Report 2002–03*, the number of wild polio cases has really shown a very significant decline: there were 1934 wild cases of polio in the country in 1998; this declined to 1264 in 1999, to 265 in 2000, and to 268 in 2001.

An independent policy to tackle the HIV/AIDS situation in the country along with a national blood policy has been drawn up, and according to the latest annual report of the MHFW, the government has put in place a 'dynamic action plan to operationalize this blood policy with significant revitalization of the existing blood transfusion services within the country'. Some 700 targeted interventions aimed at people who are at higher risk of contracting HIV are in various stages of implementation across the country and the results are beginning to show. Although there is a long way ahead, we can be confident that all is being done to keep HIV/AIDS at bay.

India is also inching towards the elimination of leprosy, and the government counts this as a major strength of its overall health programmes. This would mean a prevalence rate of less than one case for every 10,000 people. According to the MHFW, the prevalence rate for leprosy declined from 57.6 per 10,000 in 1981 to 4.2 cases per 10,000 as on 1 April 2002. There has been remarkable progress in the incidence of TB as well: 'China and India have shown remarkable progress in expanding population coverage (with Directly Observed Short-term Treatment—DOTS) while maintaining high cure rates. Some 50,000 new TB patients are put on effective therapy each month in India alone' (Brundtland and Wolfenson, 2003).

It is evident that when the government sets its sights on a clear target, it has the human resources, infrastructure and nationwide network to be able to achieve that goal. In Haryana, the panchayati raj rule book states that any villager with more than two children born after April 1995 cannot contest the panchayat election (Sahai, 2001). In Andhra Pradesh the former chief minister, N. Chandrababu Naidu, called for strict adherence to the two-child norm from 1 April 2001 by party members of the Telegu Desam. Any member who had a third child after this date would be debarred from organizational posts and nominated government posts (Sahai, 2001). Going beyond family planning, the government is also trying to work out methods of partnering with the private sector. In an innovative programme, the Karnataka State Department of Health has been sub-contracting certain non-clinical services for eighty-two secondary-level hospitals under a World Bank-funded project called the Karnataka Health Systems Development Project (KHSDP), begun as a pilot initiative in 1997 (Peters et al., 2002). Necessary maintenance jobs like cleaning the hospital and managing the waste generated were given out to private vendors, and although contract payments were lower than the salaries of cleaning staff, the cleanliness of the hospital improved.

While partnerships show strength, the challenge also lies in being able to recognize the clear roles of government and non-government institutions. In citing the experiences of Drs Abhay and Rani Bang of SEARCH (Chapter 8), it was found that SEARCH's innovative methodology to work in collaboration with the government did not succeed. SEARCH has always been clear that the roles of the voluntary sector and the government are different, and that a successful effort from an NGO will never simply duplicate a governmental effort only because the latter has failed to provide the basic facilities that it was meant to in the health sector. The real impact of an NGO shows when it creates enough pressure on the government to make sure that whatever services are provided are of a certain quality.

The MHFW now has a forward-looking health policy in

place. Since the NHP of 1983, much has changed in India's health system. For one, lifestyle diseases have become a bigger burden than they were earlier, especially heart disease, cancer and diabetes. With life expectancy having gone up considerably, there is also a greater need for infrastructure that can look after the growing populace of the elderly. These new factors have in some ways redefined the health sector and policy makers believe these factors are the ones that have created a need for review of the old policy. It is also hoped that the new policy will catalyse the formation of a structure that will help reduce inequities and allow the less-privileged sections of society better access to public health services. The earlier policy also had a laudable goal of decentralizing services, but then stopped short. There are plans to flatten out the vertical implementation structure of disease-control programmes as they are currently run. Admittedly, these are difficult to run for each disease, are more cost-intensive, and need much more human resources. The NHP of 2002 also hopes to involve homoeopaths and other alternative practitioners in the dispensation of the public health-care system across the country. This is a recognition of the fact that there is a substantial number of medical experts who are formally trained in their disciplines and can easily be roped into the mainstream if some basic hurdles can be overcome.

The First, Strong Rays of Reform

The success of the RKS in Indore soon became a model for replication across the state and the government went ahead spreading the idea to other places where people showed the right level of motivation to do similar work. Today the RKS operates across the state, it has the state minister in charge of the particular district as head, and involves government officials, doctors, the Red Cross and senior citizens of the Rotary Club. A massive number of people—anywhere between 65 and 70 million—are today benefiting from the RKS. Amazingly, the trend from public to private has been reversed and many medicos have moved from private practice to managing government hospitals under the RKS. Close to Rs 400 million have been raised by citizens in the last four years to help improve hospital care in the state. Each month, RKS societies raise anywhere between Rs 25 and 30 million. The real reasons for success are a committed officer, motivated citizens, and a supportive government. Without these it wouldn't have worked. More often than not, the government has been known to actively interfere in such self-styled reform. The government views dedicated officials with suspicion, certain that they are attempting to take the law into their own hands. As a result, officers are transferred at will. But, like Mohanty says, it is really the people who made it possible. Among his favourite examples is Binni Bai, a vegetable vendor from Raipur. She sold her land and donated Rs 10 lakh to the RKS, while she herself continues to live in a hut. The rickshaw pullers of Satna, along with small shopkeepers, donated Rs 1.5 lakh, all huge sums for such people who break their backs to be able to eat two square meals a day. One ward boy contributed Rs 25,000 to the MYH.

The RKS worked as a facilitator for people to 'give up their complacency, get them enthused and unleash their energy to participate and change the state of affairs in public hospitals,' says Mohanty. Can similar movements also help the country's most prestigious hospital, AIIMS, where patients have seen rats—even in the ICU—and where the level of motivation of its huge staff is at a low ebb? The RKS example has also exploded a popular myth: Indians want everything for free. Well, give them quality service and even the poorest of the poor will try and pay whatever possible. In fact, Mohanty feels that a small charge gives each patient the right to demand quality health care. Therefore, at a small level but with highly committed planning the Collector of Indore managed several changes that transformed the very foundations of health care. This IAS officer with a difference used his bureaucratic clout to shake up a decadent and rotting system. His methodology was simple and easy to replicate, and his logic straightforward and workable.

> The people are now in charge. They generate resources from within without depending on the government, businesses or external agencies. Now they are a crucial part of the health delivery system itself. This transition from sullen fatalism to active participation, from chaos to order and from despair to hope is what enthuses and inspires us. (Mohanty, 2001)

Each worker within the RKS never lost sight of one core value, which was to involve ordinary people in the process. In neighbouring Sri Lanka, which still has better health indices than India (Chapter 7), there is a group called Sarvodaya Shramadana. This group has identified ten very basic human needs, the most important being a clean environment, both physical and mental; enough food and clean water; education; and supply of energy resources and fuel. In villages where this programme was active the people simply worked out ways and means to meet these vital goals. Dr A.T. Ariyaratne, President of the Sarvodaya Shramadana has said: 'People's movements should not be seen as a threat by public health authorities but rather as an opportunity for constructive cooperation' (WHO, 2000a). In India, while there are many examples of how holistic community-based programmes can make a difference and bring about positive change, the relationship between the government and individuals or institutions, which have been instruments of that change, was somehow always one of animosity, with the government adopting a typical dog-in-the-manger attitude. Now, the NHP of 2002 promises change, and admits that there can be no success without the involvement of people or people-based institutions. In fact, if successful local programmes could be allowed to come to the forefront, and if the people of communities involved in these programmes could be allowed to have a stake in that success, health-care reform might move ahead much more rapidly. All the good intentions outlined in the policy can become reality if the people are actively involved in it. RKS, SEARCH, SEWA, they all echo the same. In fact, SEARCH has clearly documented how the health infrastructure proved ineffective simply because government programmes had no connection with the problems of the people they treated. The Bangs learnt this lesson early on and constantly 'SEARCH'ed the community for its unique problems. Identifying those unique problems is half the solution. But unless governments—both centre and state— are able to accept the individual successes of NGOs and also integrate those effective methodologies into their larger state- and country-level programmes, sustaining change will be difficult.

It must be said that effective and positive change has also come about because of reform in the law and legal activism (Chapter 5). Whether it is regarding the removal of a senior person in the MCI, or holding doctors accountable, or fighting for the professional rights of people living with HIV/AIDS, the courts and lawyers are doing their bit to usher in a new era in health care, where questions are asked and answers are sought, where doctors are responsible more than just in spirit for the well-being of their wards, and where health care has to be provided to all people as a fundamental right. Another ray of hope has emerged from global partnerships that have evolved over the years, partnerships that are not just occasional, dollar-churning external institutions, but that are building credible, in-country systems with Indian set-ups. The Bill and Melinda Gates Foundation works in India, trying to reach out to 7 million people who live at risk of contracting HIV/AIDS by integrating and scaling up the country's response to protection against the dreaded disease. The Global Fund to Fight AIDS, TB and Malaria is also a major new contributor in beefing up India's response to health challenges.

The country also needs to step up the collaboration between traditional knowledge systems and state-of-the-art health care. WHO has often cited the example of how Vietnam managed to tackle malaria through the development and production of artemesinin, which came from the thanh hao tree and was used as part of traditional medication. This drug is efficient against multi-drug resistant malaria and the death toll from the disease came down by a whopping 97 per cent in just five years (1992–97), with the incidence of cases also falling by 60 per cent during the same period. India, with its huge treasure trove of traditional systems and indigenous medication, can certainly improve its health structures by being more open to these systems. In fact, for many people these traditional methods are a way of life, and yet, the act of bringing these methods into mainstream health care has often been ignored, even defied. There is also the larger concern about the effective use of technology: is India using sufficient technology of the right kind to tackle its health-care problems? Health care is one sector that uses a mix of both high-end and very low-grade technologies, or no technology at all. While the value of high-tech equipments and techniques in saving life and making health better is well known, techniques like the ORS are the real marvels of health care. When *Lancet* published the research done at the International Centre for Diarrhoeal Disease Research, it declared ORS to be one of the most significant discoveries of the twentieth century (UNDP, 2001). While an intravenous drip was once the only way out, ORS showed that a simple sugar-and-salt solution did the trick, and truly revolutionized treatment for dehydration. The price differential was amazing: 10 cents for an ORS kit against at least US$ 50 for a drip for a child.

Technology has had a tangible impact on health, and there is no denying this. The *HDR, 2001* has analysed this contribution and found that in the three decades between 1960 and 1990 at least 45 per cent of the contribution towards reducing the incidence of death among children under the age of 5 was from technology. Similarly, there was a 39 per cent impact on adult female mortality, 49 per cent on adult male mortality, and 49 per cent on female life expectancy at birth. India needs to delve more deeply into similar innovative technologies and come up with workable solutions for many of its community health problems. Tropicalized vaccines that are more heat-stable and do not need stringent cold chains and maintenance have made a great difference over the years.

Reform has also begun in the sector of health finance and insurance. Although the coverage through health insurance in India remains abysmally low as far as percentage of population is concerned (it is just about 10 per cent), the opening up of the insurance market and allowing the private sector to offer insurance has had some impact. But overall, health-policy benefits are poor. What has worked are smaller experiments through self-help groups and organized cooperatives. Even so, it is a long way before out-of-pocket-expenses for treatment actually diminish, and the overall situation of financial wreckage after hospitalization is dealt with. One wonders whether this is because more than anything else, health remains a low priority: it never shows up prominently in any party's election manifesto, is reduced to background noise in many political discussions, and is ridden with a lack of understanding of the real issues involved. *The World Health Report*, 2000 has clearly set forth significant points to consider in the analysis of any health system: good government is synonymous with a healthy population and the government's responsibility for the well-being of a nation's population has to be 'continuous and permanent'; the poor—globally—are bearing the brunt of the failure of health systems to perform efficiently and to the optimum, and a large number of preventable deaths are the result of this lack of performance; a government cannot just get away with health improvement alone, it is equally responsible for making health care affordable for all, especially in countries like India where the health-care industry has grown boundlessly in the last few years. Of course, much of this growth has remained beyond the reach of ordinary Indians; the time is past when governments could ignore the private and voluntary health sectors, concentrating only on the public sector which comes directly under the health ministries of various countries. Governments will need to work towards bringing all the various aspects of total health care together for the benefit of their people; and finally, the WHO recommends not turning a blind eye to a system's failings, and not indulging in 'oversight of the entire system'. As Dr Gro Harlem Brundtland, former Director General of the WHO says in *The World Health Report*, 2000:

Whatever standards we apply, it is evident that health systems in some countries perform well, while others perform poorly. This is not due just to differences in income or expenditure: we know that performance can vary markedly, even in countries with very similar levels of health spending. The way health systems are designed, managed and financed affects people's lives and livelihoods. The difference between a well-performing health system and one that is failing can be measured in death, disability, impoverishment, humiliation and despair.

And what a difference that can make to a people and a country. The fact that a well-performing health system could mean the difference between life and death cannot be over emphasized. It is time for India to recognize this truth and address it. And the time is now.

RAISING THE SIGHTS

The World Bank was recently involved in an exhaustive exercise of analysing India's health-care system. This was a response to a felt need of the Indian government to define the kind of health system the country should have in this new century. An extensive country-wide research programme set out to explore certain basic issues—the private sector and health care, chronic disease risk factors, public and private health services and the distribution of their benefits, financial protection for health care, patient priorities, and of course the laws that guide health care in India. According to the authors of the study, more than a dozen Indian institutions, in partnership with the World Bank and the government of India, conducted the research.

It was in 1999 that the scope of this study was chalked out and a detailed research agenda emerged after intensive consultations. Studies were conducted by Indian institutions and over the next two years, the data were analysed. What has emerged could be a useful blueprint for change. Addressing the needs of India's most vulnerable people and the necessity to regularize and structure both private and public sector health care so as to make things better are two core concerns of the consultation.

The blueprint is to look after the health needs of the really poor and vulnerable sections of the population, strengthen health financing, recognize and use the positive aspects of the private sector and counter its failures to create a system that is of high quality and accountable to the people. As the authors say, 'If reforms are to be carried out in India's health sector, the vision for change must come out of the discussions among the stakeholders in the health system. Therefore, the report does not set out to prescribe detailed answers for India's future health system. It does, however, have a goal: to support informed debates and consensus building, and to help shape a health system that continually strives to be more effective, equitable, efficient, and accountable to the Indian people, and particularly to the poor' (Peters et al., 2002).

References

Introduction

Annual Report, 2002–03. New Delhi: Ministry of Health and Family Welfare, Government of India.

Encyclopaedia Brittanica and *The Hindu*, 2002. *India Book of the Year 2002*. Gurgaon: Encyclopaedia Brittanica (India) Pvt. Ltd.

Manorama Year Book, 2003. Kottayam: Malayala Manorama Co. Ltd.

National Health Policy, 2002. New Delhi: Department of Health, Ministry of Health and Family Welfare, Government of India.

National Human Rights Commission (NHRC), 1999. *Quality Assurance in Mental Health*. New Delhi: NHRC.

Reddy, Srinath K., 1998. Rising burden of cardiovascular disease in India. In *Coronary Artery Disease in India*, edited by K.K. Sethi. Kolkata: Cardiological Society of India.

UNDP, 2002. *Human Development Report*. Published for the United Nations Development Programme, New Delhi: Oxford University Press.

———, 2003. *Human Development Report*. Published for the United Nations Development Programme, New Delhi: Oxford University Press.

WHO, 2003. *Shaping the Future*. Geneva: World Health Organization.

Chapter 1

Abreu, R., and S. Menon, 1997. Return of the resilient killer. *India Today* (15 December).

Annual Report, 2002–03. New Delhi: Ministry of Health and Family Welfare, Government of India.

Banerjee, K., 1996. Emerging viral infections with special reference to India. *Indian Journal of Medical Research*, 103: 177–200.

Bhaduri, A.N., 1996. Recent outbreak of kala azar in India: Some research initiatives. In *Microbial Threats to Health in the 21st Century: Proceedings of the Second Annual Ranbaxy Science Foundation Symposium*, edited by P.L. Sharma and O.P. Sood. Amsterdam: Scientific Communications International Ltd.

Chadha, V.K., et. al., 2001. Annual risk of tuberculosis infection in Bangalore city. *Indian Journal of Tuberculosis*, 48: 63–71.

Chhabra, S.K., et. al., 1998. Prevalence of bronchial asthma in school children in Delhi. *Journal of Asthma*, 35(3): 291–96.

Chopra, R., 2001. The Indian scene. *Journal of Clinical Oncology*, 19:106–11.

Deb, S.K., 1998. Acute respiratory disease survey in Tripura in case of children below five years of age. *Journal of the Indian Medical Association*, April 96(4): 111–16.

Gaurav, R.B., and S. Kartikeyan, 2001. Levels of blood pressure in an urban community. *Bombay Hospital Journal* 43(1): 148–51.

Haq, Mahboob Ul, 1997. *Human Development in South Asia*. Human Development Centre, Karachi: Oxford University Press.

Menon, S., 1996a. Slimming centres: Weighing the pitfalls. *India Today* (15 August).

———, 1996b. Viruses: Deadly comeback. *India Today* (31 October).

————, 1997a. Killer on the prowl. *India Today* (30 June).

————, 1997b. Diabetes: Striking the young. *India Today* (24 November).

————, 1999a. Taming the demons. *India Today* (18 January).

————, 1999b. Bad news for bones. *India Today* (1 November).

————, 1999c. The clot busters. *India Today* (8 November).

Mohapatra, P.K., et al., 2001. Risk factors of malaria in the fringes of the evergreen monsoon forest of Arunachal Pradesh. *National Medical Journal* 14(3): May–June.

Nakajima, Hiroshi, 1996. Fighting disease, fostering development. Geneva: World Health Organization.

Prabhakar, R., and P.R. Narayanan, 1996. Tuberculosis in India: The continuing scourge. In *Microbial Threats to Health in the 21st Century: Proceedings of the Second Annual Ranbaxy Science Foundation Symposium*, edited by P.L. Sharma and O.P Sood. Amsterdam: Scientific Communications International Ltd.

Reddy, K.S., 1998. Global perspective on cardiovascular disease. In *Evidence Based Cardiology*, edited by S. Yusuf, J.A. Cairns, A.J. Camm, E.L. Fallen, B.J. Gersh. London: BMJ.

Ten Dam, Gerard, 1993. BCG: A partial solution. In *TB: A Global Emergency. World Health.* The Magazine of the WHO, Forty-sixth Year, No. 4, July–August.

WHO, 1996. *The World Health Report: Fighting Disease, Fostering Development.* Geneva: World Health Organization.

————, 1998a. *Emerging Infectious Diseases in South East Asia: 50 Years Commemorative Series—4.* New Delhi: Regional Office for Southeast Asia.

————, 1998b. *Tuberculosis in the Southeast Asian Region: 50 Years Commemorative Series—4.* New Delhi: Regional Office for Southeast Asia.

Chapter 2

Banerjee, N., et al., 2001. Factors determining the occurrence of unwanted pregnancies. *National Medical Journal*, 14(4): 211–12 (July–August).

Census of India, 2001. New Delhi: Government of India.

Duggal, R., and S. Amin, 1989. *Cost of Health Care*. Bombay: Foundation for Research in Community Health.

International Institute for Population Sciences and ORC Macro, 2000. *National Family Health Survey (NFHS-2), 1998–99*. Printed in New Delhi for the International Institute for Population Sciences, Mumbai.

Iyer, A., 1998. *Women's Reproductive Health—CEHAT*. New Delhi: Voluntary Health Association of India.

UNDP, 2002. *Human Development Report*. Published for the United Nations Development Programme. New Delhi: Oxford University Press.

UNICEF, 1996. *The Situation of Women and Children*. New Delhi: Oxford University Press.

———, 1998. *The State of the World's Children*, New York: Oxford University Press.

VHAI, 1997. *Report of the Independent Commission on Health in India*. New Delhi: Voluntary Health Association of India.

World Bank, 1996. *Improving Women's Health in India*. Directions in Development Series. Washington DC: World Bank.

Chapter 3

Annual Report, 2002–03. New Delhi: Ministry of Health and Family Welfare, Government of India.

Brundtland, Gro Harlem, 2001. *Mental Health: New Understanding, New Hope*. Geneva: World Health Organization.

ICMR, 1998. Neuroepidemiological survey in urban and rural

areas: A prevalence study. Report of an ICMR Task Force Study. New Delhi: Indian Council of Medical Research.

———, 2001. Developments in mental health scenario: Need to stop exclusion—Dare to Care. *ICMR Bulletin*, 31(4), April.

Kannan, Ramya, 2002. *India Book of the Year 2002*. Gurgaon: Encyclopaedia Brittanica (India) Pvt. Ltd.

Menon, S., 2001. Killer fire pushes India's mental asylums to reform. *Reuters Health* (7 August).

NHRC, 1999. *Quality Assurance in Mental Health*. New Delhi: National Human Rights Commission.

Reddy, M.V., and C.R. Chandrashekhar, 1998. Prevalence of mental and behavioural disorders in India. *Indian Journal of Psychiatry*, 40: 149.

WHO, 2000. *The World Health Report: Health Systems, Improving Performance*. Geneva: World Health Organization.

———, 2001. *Mental Health: New Understanding, New Hope*. Geneva: World Health Organization.

Chapter 4

Annual Report, 2002–03. New Delhi: Ministry of Health and Family Welfare, Government of India.

Duggal, R., 2001. *Utilisation of Health Services in India*. National Consultation on Health Security in India Proceedings. Organized by the Institute of Human Development and UNDP with support from the Ministry for Health and Family Welfare, Government of India.

Menon, S., 1998. Poisonous network. *India Today* (14 September).

———, 2000. Back to Dandi. *India Today* (June)

National Health Policy, 2002. New Delhi: Department of Health, Ministry of Health and Family Welfare, Government of India.

Pallikadavath, Saseendran, and R. William Stones, 2001. *Women's Reproductive Health Security in the Wake of the*

HIV/AIDS Epidemic in India. National Consultation on Health Security in India Proceedings. Organized by the Institute of Human Development and UNDP with support from the Ministry for Health and Family Welfare, Government of India.

Peters, D.H., et. al., 2002. *Better Health Systems for India's Poor—Findings, Analysis and Options*. Washington DC, USA: Human Development Network, The World Bank.

Ravi Kanth, D., 2003. WHO concerned about polio spread in India. *Deccan Herald* (13 May).

Seetha Prabhu, K., and V. Selvaraju, 2001. *Public Financing for Health Security in India: Issues and Trends*. National Consultation on Health Security in India Proceedings. Organized by the Institute of Human Development and UNDP with support from the Ministry for Health and Family Welfare, Government of India.

WHO, 2000. *The World Health Report: Health Systems, Improving Performance*. Geneva: World Health Organization.

World Bank, 2001. *World Development Report, 2000–01, Attacking Poverty: Opportunity, Empowerment and Security*. Washington DC, USA: Oxford University Press, for the International Bank for Reconstruction and Development.

Chapter 5

Baru, Rama V., 2001. *Privatisation of Health Care and its Implications for Health Security*. National Consultation on Health Security Proceedings. Organized by the Institute for Human Development and UNDP with support from the Ministry of Health and Family Welfare, Government of India.

DSPRUD, 1999. *Promotion of Rational Use of Drugs in the Indian Scenario: A WHO–India Initiative*. New Delhi: Delhi Society for Promotion of Rational Use of Drugs.

Duggal, R., 2001. *Utilisation of Health Services in India*. National Consultation on Health Security Proceedings. Organized by the Institute for Human Development and UNDP with support from the Ministry of Health and Family Welfare, Government of India.

Economic Survey 1999–2000. New Delhi: Ministry of Finance, Government of India.

Gumber, A. and V. Kulkarni, 2001. *Health Security for Workers: The Case of the Informal Sector*. National Consultation on Health Security Proceedings. Organized by the Institute for Human Development and UNDP with support from the Ministry of Health and Family Welfare, Government of India.

Indian Express, 2001. 38 partially blinded due to 'adulterated solution'. Express News Service (28 July).

Menon, S., 1997. Quacks in the box. *India Today* (20 October).

National Health Policy, 2002, New Delhi: Government of India, Department of Health, Ministry of Health and Family Welfare.

Peters, D.H., et al., 2002. *Better Health Systems for India's Poor— Findings, Analysis and Options*. Washington DC, USA: Human Development Network, The World Bank.

Seetha Prabhu, K., and V. Selvaraju, 2001. *Public Financing for Health Security in India: Issues and Trends*. National Consultation on Health Security Proceedings. Organized by the Institute for Human Development and UNDP with support from the Ministry of Health and Family Welfare, Government of India.

Thapa, V.J., and S. Menon, 2000. Growing distrust. *India Today* (25 September).

WHO, 2000. *The World Health Report: Health Systems, Improving Performance*. Geneva: World Health Organization.

World Bank, 2001. *India—Raising the Sights. Better Health Systems for India's Poor*. Washington DC, USA: Human Development Network, The World Bank.

Chapter 6

Commission on Intellectual Property Rights, 2002. *Integrating Intellectual Property Rights and Development Policy*. London.

DSPRUD, 1999. *Promotion of Rational Use of Drugs in the Indian Scenario: A WHO–India Initiative*. New Delhi: Delhi Society for Promotion of Rational Use of Drugs.

Pabrai, P.R., 2001. Quality assurance of drugs. In *The Medicines Scenario in India: Perceptions and Perspectives*, edited by A. Banerji. New Delhi: Delhi Society for Promotion of Rational Use of Drugs.

Parameswar, R., 2001. Procurement and distribution of drugs. In *The Medicines Scenario in India: Perceptions and Perspectives*, edited by A. Banerji. New Delhi: Delhi Society for Promotion of Rational Use of Drugs.

Sheth, P.D., 2001. Strengths and weaknesses of the pharmaceutical industry—A review. In *The Medicines Scenario in India: Perceptions and Perspectives*, edited by A. Banerji. New Delhi: Delhi Society for Promotion of Rational Use of Drugs.

VHAI, 1997. *Report of the Independent Commission on Health in India*. New Delhi: Voluntary Health Association of India.

WHO, 2000. *Public Health in Southeast Asia in the 21st Century*. Report and Recommendations of the Regional Conference, Calcutta, 22–24 November. New Delhi: Regional Office for Southeast Asia.

Chapter 7

National Human Development Report (NHDR), 2001. New Delhi: Planning Commission, Government of India.

Peters, D.H., et. al., 2002. *Better Health Systems for India's Poor—Findings, Analysis and Options*. Washington DC, USA: Human Development Network, The World Bank.

Planning Commission, 2002. *Report of the Committee on India*

Vision 2020. New Delhi: Government of India (under the Chairmanship of S.P. Gupta).

UNDP, 2003. *Human Development Report*. Published for the United Nations Development Programme, New Delhi: Oxford University Press.

Chapter 8

Census of India, 2001. New Delhi: Government of India.

Duggal, R., 2001. *Utilisation of Health Care Services in India*. National Consultation on Health Security in India Proceedings. Organized by the Institute of Human Development and UNDP with support from the Ministry for Health and Family Welfare, Government of India.

National Human Development Report, 2001. New Delhi: Planning Commission, Government of India.

National Sample Survey, 1995–96, 52nd Round. New Delhi: National Sample Survey Organization, Department of Statistics, Government of India.

Shariff, Abusaleh, 1999. *India: Human Development Report—A Profile of Indian States in the 1990s*. New Delhi: National Council of Applied Economic Research.

VHAI, 1991. *Anubhav—Experiences in Health and Community Development: Vivekananda Girijana Kalyana Kendra*. New Delhi: Voluntary Health Association of India.

———, 1997. *Report of the Independent Commission on Health*. New Delhi: Voluntary Health Association of India.

———, 1998. *Anubhav—Experiences in Health and Community Development: SEARCH*. New Delhi: Voluntary Health Association of India.

Chapter 9

Brundtland, G.H., and J.D. Wolfenson, 2003. Fighting TB Worldwide. *The Hindu* (11 April).

Chatterjee, Mirai. My health: My asset and my right—A case study of the Self-Employed Women's Association in Gujarat, India, <http://www.sewa.org>.

Jana, Samarjit, et al., 1999. Creating an enabling environment: Lessons learnt from the Sonagachi Project, India. In *Research for Sex Work 2*. Amsterdam, The Netherlands: VU Medical Centre.

Kannan, K.P., et al., 1991. *Health and Development in Rural Kerala*. Kerala Sastra Sahitya Parishad.

Mohanty, S.R., 2001. *Management of Public Hospitals through People's Participation: The Case of the Rogi Kalyan Samiti*. National Consultation on Health Security in India Proceedings. Organized by the Institute for Human Development and UNDP with support from the Ministry of Health and Family Welfare, Government of India.

Panchamukhi, P.R., and N. Nayak, 2001. *Health Security for the Poor: Health Insurance through Health Care Cooperative*. National Consultation on Health Security in India Proceedings. Organized by the Institute for Human Development and UNDP with support from the Ministry of Health and Family Welfare, New Delhi.

Peters, D.H., et al., 2002. *Better Health Systems for India's Poor—Findings, Analysis and Options*. Washington DC, USA: Human Development Network, The World Bank.

Sahai, Nandini, 2001. Want to be a sarpanch? Hide your third child. *People* 2(1), January.

UNDP, 2001. *Human Development Report*. Published for the United Nations Development Programme, New Delhi: Oxford University Press.

VHAI, 1997. *Report of the Independent Commission on Health in India*. New Delhi: Voluntary Health Association of India.

———, 1999. *Anubhav—Kerala Shastra Sahitya Parishad*. New Delhi: Voluntary Health Association of India.

WHO, 2000a. *Public Health in Southeast Asia in the 21ˢᵗ Century*. Report and Recommendations of the Regional Conference, Calcutta, 22–24 November 1999. New Delhi: Regional Office for Southeast Asia.

———, 2000b. *The World Health Report: Health Systems, Improving Performance*. Geneva: World Health Organization.